WALKING
THE CROOKED MILE

*A Self-Help Program For Adult
Survivors of Childhood Abuse*

LINDA S. SCHRITT, R.S.W.

TRAFFORD
PUBLISHING

Note for Librarians: A cataloguing record for this book is available from Library and Archives Canada at www.collectionscanada.ca/amicus/index-e.html

ISBN 1-4120-7542-4

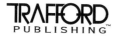

Printed in Victoria, BC, Canada. Printed on paper with minimum 30% recycled fibre. Trafford's print shop runs on "green energy" from solar, wind and other environmentally-friendly power sources.

TRAFFORD
PUBLISHING™

Offices in Canada, USA, Ireland and UK

This book was published *on-demand* in cooperation with Trafford Publishing. On-demand publishing is a unique process and service of making a book available for retail sale to the public taking advantage of on-demand manufacturing and Internet marketing. On-demand publishing includes promotions, retail sales, manufacturing, order fulfilment, accounting and collecting royalties on behalf of the author.

Book sales for North America and international:

Trafford Publishing, 6E–2333 Government St.,
Victoria, BC V8T 4P4 CANADA

phone 250 383 6864 (toll-free 1 888 232 4444)

fax 250 383 6804; email to orders@trafford.com

Book sales in Europe:

Trafford Publishing (UK) Limited, 9 Park End Street, 2nd Floor
Oxford, UK OX1 1HH UNITED KINGDOM

phone 44 (0)1865 722 113 (local rate 0845 230 9601)

facsimile 44 (0)1865 722 868; info.uk@trafford.com

Order online at:

trafford.com/05-2437

14 13 12

In Memory of My Dad, Roy Cyril Thompson.
A man who gave friendship and compassion
to those that others did not see.

There is a place within me where I exist.
Uncorrupted by touch or whispered word.
It is the place God made for me
when He called me into being.
It is there I am His creation
not the creation of the world.
It is the place I will return to
when I learn the Truth.
It is the place where I will be free
to know and be who I am.

It is my spirit.

CONTENTS

PART I BUILDING A FOUNDATION FOR HEALING

PART II RECLAIMING YOURSELF

INTRODUCTION

There was a crooked man who walked a crooked mile. He found a crooked sixpence upon a crooked stile. He bought a crooked cat who caught a crooked mouse. And they all lived together in a little crooked house...

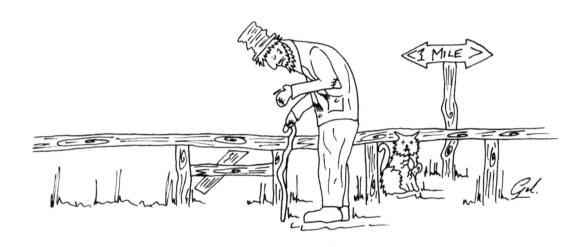

The story might have ended there if a doctor had not moved into the house next door. One day the doctor asked the crooked man, "Why do you walk all bent over like that?"

The crooked man was startled and more than a little nervous. People usually did not talk to him. In fact most people acted like they didn't see him at all. At first he just shrugged and looked at the ground. The crooked man waited for the doctor to walk away. But the doctor only repeated his question. "Isn't it obvious?" the crooked man finally said in a shaky voice. "I thought everyone could see.... I have no spine."

"Of course you have a spine," the doctor replied.

"No, you are mistaken. I am certain I do not.' The crooked man looked puzzled; this doctor was a strange fellow indeed. Perhaps he was even stranger than the crooked man himself. "I have it on very good authority. My father always told me I was 'spineless' and he was never wrong."

The doctor shook his head sadly. He had been a healer for many years and had seen this kind of thing many times before. Once he had treated a man who was 'brainless' and a woman who had spent her entire life waiting to die because she should 'never have been born.' "Your father was wrong," the doctor said kindly. "It is not that you have no spine but your spirit and your heart have been broken."

The crooked man was very surprised by the doctor's words. "What do you mean?" he cried, "my spirit and my heart are broken?" How can that be?"

"It comes from a lifetime of carrying the burden of your father's words upon your back. That is something you can change and I will help you if you let me." The doctor's eyes were full of compassion as he looked at the trembling man before him.

The crooked man was skeptical at first. He did not understand why the doctor wanted to help him, no one ever had before. The idea that his father may have been wrong was scary and exciting, all at the same time. If his father was wrong about this perhaps he had been wrong about other things he had told the crooked man. Things that had made the crooked man feel bad and stupid all his life. Although he was frightened the crooked man decided to let the doctor help him for the pain in him was becoming harder to bear. Everyday he did the exercises the doctor gave him. Some days he had new feelings in his body and his heart. Some days he felt like quitting because the ache that filled his being felt overwhelming. But the crooked man persevered and gradually his bent back grew straighter. After a time he realized his eyes were no longer always looking at the ground. At first he was too frightened to do more than to glance cautiously around for he had spent his whole life seeing only what stood a few feet in front of him. Over time he came to realize there was great beauty in the world and he even stopped being so afraid of people. He could see now who they were but more importantly he was learning who he was. He was a man like all other men with strengths and weaknesses. He did some things right and some things wrong. He could make mistakes and learn from them. He could choose what to believe and what not to believe. He could look at his reflection and smile. He stopped hearing his father's voice and heard his own instead. The crooked man stopped being ashamed.

The man no longer walked the crooked mile for there was much for him to see and do. Now he rides a shiny red bicycle everywhere he goes.

—ɯ—

Every person who has been abused has walked their own crooked mile carrying their abuser on their back. We were not created with 'crookedness' but abuse fills us with twists and turns which lead us through frightening landscapes of false beliefs. Your life is distorted, off balance to some degree. Your world is filtered through the abuse. You must raise your eyes and see yourself and the world around you as you really are. We free ourselves of the lies through healing the wounds within our hearts and our spirits. Understanding the impact of abuse straightens out the crooked road and makes it a straight, clear path to healing.

Healing is a process. Webster defines a process as a *continuous action or series of actions that lead to the accomplishment of a result.* By building a solid foundation of knowledge you will get good results in your healing process. If you want your house to stand firm you don't build it on shaky ground. The knowledge you acquire as you work through this book will support you in developing understanding, self-awareness and the acknowledgement of truth. *The truth will set you free.*

This book was written to free you from living a 'crooked' life, a life that is not yours, and to live instead the life you were created for. It is a tool to help you identify the distortions and faulty beliefs which developed as a result of the abuse you suffered. The book is divided into two parts. Part I provides information which will support you in building your foundation for healing and then personalizing it so it is meaningful and relevant to you. The information given is fundamental, intended to give you a general working knowledge of the impact of abuse. A list of recommended readings is provided if you wish to explore the concepts in greater depth. I encourage you to do so, knowledge is power.

Part II is designed to assist you in reclaiming yourself, recovering the parts of self that have been lost. Taking control of your life means taking responsibility for your own well being. Part II will lead you step by step through the process of developing your personal power. To claim your power you must come into full awareness of your feelings, where they originate from and how they influence you in your daily life. Only then can you truly begin to *live* your life instead of just *surviving* it.

This is a simple text. It is a compilation of ideas, personal and professional experience, several theoretical perspectives and a healthy dose of commonsense. Most of the personal comments included are not direct quotes from one individual but rather a combination of many voices brought together as one in an expression of their common experience. My goal is to present the information as clearly and concisely as possible. I wrote this book because I have absolute faith in the resilience of the human spirit. No matter what has happened in your life within you lies the strength and the wisdom to reclaim your true self, the person you were created to be.

I can't emphasize enough the importance of doing *all* the writing exercises. It is an essential part of your healing process. Writing things down gives you the awareness and clarity necessary to see the *truth*. The purpose of this book is to help you live the truth. *Abuse is something that happened to you but it doesn't have to define who you are.* It is time to stop living the lie.

"We (abuse victims) live in a world of secret places where emotional beatings and lies are the norm and kindness is a rarity. This dark prison is our spirit, battered and broken by our abusers. The bars that hold us captive are fear and shame. I plan on making a prison break and running out into the sunshine. I will not do this quietly. I plan on yelling, 'I love you and I forgive you' in a loud strong voice. I plan on saying this to myself and meaning it. I know now it was not my fault and it was not my shame. I plan on being free." - L

—⚭—

Abuse is a lie. Through the abusive words and actions of others many of you have come to believe you have no worth and no one could possibly love you if they knew who you really were. This is a lie. Each of us comes into this world deserving of love and respect simply because we exist. We exist because we were meant to be. No one is here by random chance. **We are all planned creations of the Creator.** We all arrive with the same capacity to give and receive love. It is through this giving and receiving that we enter into our humanity. The child who is born into an abusive environment is no less deserving than the child who is fortunate enough to be born into a loving home. The child who is molested is no less deserving of love and protection than the child who is not. The child who is disregarded is no less precious than the child who is cherished. Those of you who have been abused were not responsible for the abusive actions inflicted upon you, no matter what you may have been told.

As children we used to play a game called 'Pass it On.' The object of the game was to whisper a message to the person next to you and pass it on down the line. The last person would repeat out loud what they had heard. Of course the end result was distorted, bearing little or no resemblance to what the true message was. Many of you are still playing 'Pass it On.'

The true message of the abuser is: *"I am a …..frightened…..angry…..insecure… out of control…..person who refuses to accept responsibility for my own life and my own pain so I will pass it on to you so you can carry it for me."*

The distorted message the victim hears is: *"There must be something about me that caused this to happen. If I weren't so…..bad…..stupid-…..ugly…..no good…..it wouldn't have happened. It must be my fault. I don't deserve anything better. No one could ever really love me if they knew what I was really like."*

—⚭—

The longer the messages play the more distorted they become. Your life filters through these messages. Your feelings, thoughts and behaviors all reflect these distorted messages. You stoop and bend and twist yourself trying to accommodate this way of *being* in the world. You begin to "Walk the Crooked Mile"

"My mother always compared me to my sister who she thought was perfect. No matter how hard I tried it seemed like it was never good enough to gain her recognition or approval. No matter how much success I have achieved as an adult I still have a hard time accepting that I am as good as other people. Even when I'm told what a good job I've done I suspect people are only trying to be nice. I try to do what other people want and expect of me even if I don't want to. I'm afraid if I don't no one will want me around any more."

It is within your power to stop living the lies of abuse and enter fully into reality, the truth of who you are. It is within your power to start living the life you were meant to have. A life that is full of what God intended when He called you into being, to work with purpose, to learn, to have joy and take satisfaction in everyday tasks, to give and receive love and to know the world is a better place because you are in it.

Personalize:

Take a few minutes to write down your thoughts and feelings as you begin your healing process.

_____

_____

_____

_____

_____

_____

_____

PART I

Building A Foundation For Healing

UNDERSTANDING WHAT ABUSE IS

Statistics suggest that millions of adults are victims of childhood abuse. Yet there remains a great deal of confusion about what constitutes abuse.

"I was emotionally abused by my husband for years without realizing what it was. I thought he was trying to make me a better person with his constant fault finding. I told myself I was being too sensitive, he didn't mean to be hurtful. Now I know he was beating me up day after day with his words. He turned out to be just like my father."

Personalize:

Write down your definition of abuse as it is right now.

_____

_____

_____

_____

_____

_____

_____

The Oxford dictionary defines abuse as:

abuse, 1. A misuse. 2. An unjust or corrupt practice. 3. Abusive words or insults.

abused, abusing 1. To make a bad or wrong use of, to abuse one's authority.

2. To treat badly. 3. To attack in words, to utter insults to or about.

There is a common misconception that abuse is primarily a problem of the poorly educated and low income members of our society. In truth; abuse is an equal opportunity affliction that knows no socio-economic boundaries. Anyone can be abused, anyone can be an abuser.

There are three broad categories of abuse: *physical, emotional and sexual.* Any form of abuse impedes healthy emotional development. It denies the victim the security that comes from knowing the world is basically safe and they have power and influence in their own lives. These are essential elements for a psychologically, emotionally and spiritually satisfying life. Although each of the three types of abuse trauma has its own fingerprint, all adversely influence:

- The capacity to allow oneself to know and to be known by another, which is the definition of true emotional intimacy.

- The ability to identify accurately the emotions of self and others and respond appropriately.

- The ability to function effectively and with influence in their various environments.

- The development of positive self-image.

All forms of abuse evolve from issues of control. The abuser finds a means of exerting power over the victim. Intimidation and indifference are the universal weapons of the abuser. These are wielded with little or no empathy for the victim. Abusers may or may not be aware of the impact of their actions. They are often so focused on their own self-gratification and self-protection they feel justified in what they do. A good example is the parent who physically beats his child saying, "*That's what my dad did to me and I turned out alright.*" Thus the abuser continues to protect himself from his own repressed feelings of pain and powerlessness by acting them out on his victim. The abuser blames the victim for their own pain.

"I wouldn't have to hit you if you would just listen."

"If you would get better grades I would spend more time with you."

"If you keep bugging me about your feelings I'm never going to listen."

PHYSICAL ABUSE

Physical abuse can be defined as any *deliberate act* which results in physical injury to another. Physical abuse includes pushing, shoving, punching, slapping, kicking, scratching, biting, pinching, burning, smothering and poisoning. Physical abuse can begin while the child is still in the womb through the mother's use of drugs and/or alcohol. Children and adults also suffer physical abuse through acts of neglect. Inadequate food, shelter, clothing, medical care and safe environments are all forms of physical neglect.

"I remember well the lessons of my childhood. They are burned into my body and my brain. I learned to watch, to listen, to be silent in the face of the storm that was you. I learned the sound a hand makes on a face and a fist makes on a body. I learned to say I'm sorry for things I didn't even understand the wrongness of. I learned the best places to hide from you and from my feelings. You told me someday I would thank you for making me a man. I learned to be what you called a man but I never learned to be myself or knew who I even was. Yes, you taught me lessons I won't forget but I will never thank you for them."

EMOTIONAL ABUSE

Emotional abuse is the form of maltreatment which denies the fulfillment of our psychological needs. Emotional abuse is the companion of all other forms of abuse. Any relationship that lacks empathy (understanding the other person's feelings) cannot fail to be emotionally abusive. Healthy relationships demonstrate a strong desire to understand others as well as concern for their well-being. As human beings we need to be loved, accepted, heard and understood. Being ridiculed, verbally assaulted and having our thoughts and feeling disregarded and ignored is emotionally devastating. *Sticks and stones* can break your bones but words can break your heart. Words hurt; those which are spoken and those which are not. Never or seldom hearing anything that makes you feel accepted and cared for is painful, it is emotional neglect. Witnessing abuse is another form of emotional abuse. It is particularly damaging when children witness spousal abuse. Children who observe one parent physically or verbally battering the other experience deep emotional trauma.

Emotional abuse is epidemic in our culture, in our homes, in our schools and workplaces. We seriously underestimate the damage sustained by being emotionally abused. Unless it occurs in conjunction with another form of abuse emotional maltreatment is often overlooked or minimized. Emotional abuse is, in my estimation, the most prevalent and untreated form of abuse.

In my work as an abuse counselor I often hear statements disclosing emotional abuse prefaced with:

"I know this is stupid but…."
"I know I'm overreacting but…."
"I guess I'm just being a baby but…."

It is not stupid, childish or an overreaction to feel and express pain that is inflicted on you emotionally. It is real, legitimate and must be validated.

"It is the invisible wounds that cause me the most pain. There were so many times I tried to tell my husband how hurt I was over something he said only to be told I was wrong…about what I said…about how I felt…about what I wanted. If I tried to defend myself it only made things worse. By the time he was done telling me what was wrong with me I would be numb with pain and full of self doubt. It took a long time for me to realize that I wasn't causing my own pain, my husband was. I think it made him feel powerful to hurt me. In fact he was doing exactly what my father had done."

"I know my mother thinks she is being helpful when she comments on my appearance, my relationships and everything she thinks I could improve upon, which is just about everything. The truth is it is not helpful at all. She has done this to me all my life and I still feel exactly the same way… worthless, like nothing I am or I do will ever be good enough."

"I'm sick of my parents fighting all the time. Sometimes my mom comes into my room crying. I feel sorry for her but it makes me mad too. I'm tired of trying to deal with their crap. I'M THE KID THEY'RE THE PARENTS!"

SEXUAL ABUSE

Sexual abuse can be the most emotionally devastating of all forms of abuse. It violates all aspects of the self, emotionally, physically and spiritually. No part of the victim is left untouched. Innocence is lost and shame is its replacement.

Sexual abuse occurs when one person uses another for sexual gratification. Any time an individual, adult or child is physically or psychologically over powered sexual abuse has occurred. Many victims of sexual abuse believe they consented if physical force was not used. This is not true. Psychological manipulation is as powerful as physical force.

There are two categories of sexual abuse:

Active:

This includes all sexual activity which involves physical contact.

- vaginal and anal intercourse or penetration with an object or finger
- being fondled or being forced to fondle another
- being forced to engage in acts of oral sex
- being kisses or stroked in a sexual manner

Passive:

This includes all activity that doesn't involve physical contact.

- Being forced to look at or pose for pornographic material
- Being forced to look at sexual body parts or sexual acts
- Inappropriate remarks about sexual body parts
- Voyeurism

Children who have been abused loose their childhood and their innocence. They no longer have the opportunity to develop as sexual beings at their own pace, they become sexualized instead. The impact of sexualization can be seen in:

- Confusion about sexual identity and normal sexual behavior. This is often demonstrated by obsessive sexual preoccupation and behavior.

"I get these feelings about some of my male friends. I don't know whether that means I'm gay or not. My uncle used to call me a little fag because I was embarrassed by the dirty magazines and movies he made me watch when he babysat. I sleep with a lot of women but lately I've started going into gay porn sites on the net. It seems like I think about this stuff all the time."

- Confusion of sex with love and non-sexual needs. This is often demonstrated through promiscuous, seductive and/or aggressive sexual behavior.

"I was called a slut all through school. I guess I was. At first I just slept with guys who were nice to me but after awhile it was pretty much anyone who wanted to. I knew they just wanted to get laid but I liked the feeling of being wanted even if it was just for a few minutes."

- Aversion to sex and intimacy. This is often demonstrated by avoidance of or anxious reactions to sexual intimacy.

"I'm married to a great guy but I'm afraid he is going to end up leaving me. I really hate having sex and I know he is getting fed up. Whenever he touches me I just freeze up. I force myself when I can't think of an excuse to get out of it. He keeps asking what is wrong. He is starting to think I don't love him. I can't tell him what my father did to me. I'm afraid he would be so disgusted he would never want to see me again."

Personalize:

Has your definition of abuse changed? If yes, in what way?

_____

_____

_____

_____

_____

_____

_____

_____

FUNDAMENTAL RIGHTS

The right to be safe from physical or emotional harm

The right to your own identity

The right to have the consideration of others

The right to be treated with respect

The right to express yourself

All human beings have fundamental rights. All forms of abuse violate your rights.

Understanding the Impact of Abuse

"The truth about our childhood is stored up in our body and although we repress it, we can never alter it. Our intellect can be deceived, our feelings manipulated, our perceptions confused and our bodies tricked with medications. But someday the body will present its bill, for it is incorruptible as a child who, still whole in spirit, will accept no compromises or excuses, and will not stop tormenting us until we stop evading the truth." Alice Miller, Thou Shalt Not Be Aware. P.19

Working through the healing process has been compared to peeling the layers off an onion. I like this analogy because it gives you a visual picture of the process, peeling away the layers of distortion and finally crying, giving voice to the suffering child who lives within you.

To understand the impact of abuse there are two key points that must be remembered:

1. Trauma continues after abuse ends.

2. The body stores memory not only in our brain, or cognitive memory, but also in the form of feelings and physical sensations. These remain present even in the event that there are no cognitive memories. Memories are stored at the age the abusive incident occurred.

During adulthood memory or *truth* may begin to emerge in fragmented pieces. These fragmented memories can be triggered by anything consciously or unconsciously associated with the abuse. The memories may emerge in the form of feelings or body sensations rather than thought. The victim may be overwhelmed with feelings of terror, powerlessness or dread which they can't explain. They may experience physical pain, strange body sensations, hear sounds or have vague visual impressions. The feelings attached to these emerging memories will be experienced exactly as they were felt at the time the abuse occurred. If the victim is unable to attach their present feeling to the past abuse they will inevitably attach it to something in the present. It is important to note that even in situations where the victim has a cognitive memory of the abuse it is not unusual for them not to connect their current feelings and behaviors to the abusive event.

For example an adult who was sexually abused at the age of four will feel the fear and confusion of the four year old child.

"It started after the birth of my daughter. For no reason I would feel like I couldn't breathe. I had a hard time swallowing and was afraid I was going to choke. I began eating only soft foods. I'd get weird feelings whenever I ate. I became paranoid and started thinking that someone was trying to poison me. At meal time I would wait until someone else tasted the food first before I would eat it. I knew my behavior was not normal but I couldn't stop the feelings no matter what I told myself. I became so consumed with fear I was afraid to go out. I thought I was going crazy."

The birth of the victim's daughter triggered suppressed memories of being sexually assaulted. At the age of four the victim had been forced to perform oral sex on her perpetrator. Initially these memories emerged in body sensations and feelings. Because the victim didn't understand what was happening to her she became increasingly anxious and fearful. The anxiety eventually escalated to full blown panic attacks. These attacks terrified her. She felt she was losing control of herself and her life. To cope she began to avoid any situation that might trigger a panic attack. She became increasingly fearful around unfamiliar people and environments. The victim's life began to revolve around being *safe*.

With the assistance of a counselor the victim eventually reclaimed memories of the assault. She remembered choking on the perpetrator's semen and wondering if it was poison. Unfortunately by the time she made the connection between the sexual abuse and what she was feeling in the present the victim had developed irrational fears and obsessive tendencies. Her self-esteem, the quality of her life and her relationships were damaged. In this manner the trauma continued and was actually magnified long after the abusive incident was over.

Preparing to Heal / Self-Care

We are all unique beings with our own individual heart, mind, body and spirit. Although as an abuse survivor you share certain commonalities there is no generic road map that will lead you to your place of healing. You must find your own points of reference. Life circumstance, the nature of the abuse and support systems are some of the factors I will be referring to. These reference points bring personal meaning and awareness to your experiences and how you have been impacted by them. No matter how confused your thoughts and feelings are right now you do possess the right answers for yourself. The healing process for each person is uniquely their own. It will progress in its own time, in its own way. For some of you it will be necessary to remember the details of your abuse for others it is simply enough to know that you have been abused. I believe we remember only what is necessary to heal. Healing is not an easy journey but it is far more difficult to continue living the lie.

You are fighting to regain your life. No one would consider going into battle without first making preparations. I urge you before you begin the healing process to do the same. Your enemy is the lie of abuse. It has had a stronghold in your life for a long time, it may not surrender easily but if you are determined in your intention to heal it will surrender.

As you begin your healing process I strongly encourage you to treat yourself with love and consideration. Hold your head up high and respect yourself for your strength, your determination and your honesty.

SELF-CARE

The following are some simple steps that you can take to nurture and support your emotional well-being throughout this process.

- Remember that you have already survived the abuse. No matter how intense the memories, or the feelings attached to the memories are, you have already survived the events. Every day remind yourself of this and congratulate yourself for your strength.

- Many survivors express the most difficult and frightening of all their feelings to deal with is anger. As you become aware of the numerous ways you've been effected by the abuse you may feel overwhelming rage. It can be very tempting to repress those feelings but expressing your anger is an important part of your recovery. Laura Davis and Ellen Bass in their groundbreaking book, *The Courage to Heal*, refer to anger as "the backbone of healing." Anger is a natural, healthy response to abuse. Allowing yourself to express anger is a way of saying what happened to you was not okay. The key in dealing with your anger is to release it in appropriate and constructive ways and directing it to where it belongs.

- If you feel overwhelmed consider finding a professional counselor who can assist and support you through the recovery process. I strongly recommend this. As you move into greater awareness it is not unusual to be flooded with intense feelings and physical sensations. Remember, memories are stored in the mind and the body at the age they occurred. If you experience feelings such as powerlessness this doesn't mean you are powerless in the present but rather how you felt at the time the abuse occurred. These feelings have been brought forth into the present. It can be very helpful, at these times to have a counselor assist you in understanding and dealing with your feelings as they emerge.

- Don't push yourself beyond your limits of tolerance. A child who is afraid of the dark will not overcome the fear by being left alone in a dark room. If pushed too quickly the fear only becomes more intense. The child must be able to maintain a tolerable level of anxiety. To conquer the fear will be a gradual process, first leaving a hall light on, then a night light and so on until the dark is no longer threatening and fearful. You must do the same. Remember to treat yourself gently as you enter your own dark places of pain. Respect and honor yourself and your process. It will take as long as it needs to take.

- Get your allies in place. If there are people you can trust and rely on for support let them know you may need to call them. If you don't feel comfortable disclosing your abuse simply state you are dealing with some old issues. If anyone pressures you to be more specific they are not respecting your boundaries and therefore are not the kind of support person you need. Be clear in what you need from your supports; a shoulder to cry on or perhaps some form of distraction to give yourself an emotional break. If you don't know individuals who can serve as supports consider help lines and/or support groups. If you are able to do this you have already taken a big step in the right direction. To trust and ask for help doesn't typically come easy for abuse survivors.

LANGUAGE:

Imagine taking a trip to a foreign country and not speaking the language. You might manage basic communications but it would be especially difficult to give clear, exact information about who you are and what you need. The healing process can be likened to taking such a trip. You are venturing into unchartered territory and are understandably anxious. To successfully navigate this journey it will be especially helpful to speak the language. Using precise language helps us to develop clarity in our thoughts, feelings and communications. Many abuse victims learned early in life it was unsafe to express emotion or, for that manner, even feel emotion and consequently have a limited emotional vocabulary. Identifying and communicating our feelings gives us valuable insights into our inherent personality traits (the character we are born with). It is especially important for children to be able to express themselves if they are to succeed in developing a healthy self-image. Unfortunately expression of self is not an option for many abuse victims.

"Anytime I tried to talk about my feelings I always ended up being laughed at and told I was too sensitive. It was easier to pretend everything was fine. As an adult I have a hard time knowing what I feel. I have been told I am a chameleon, taking on the opinions of whoever is around me."

Personalize:

To assist you in the identification of your feelings and personality traits the following vocabulary lists have been included to help you. These lists have been organized into primary feeling states and personality traits. The specific feelings you experience create the overall primary feeling state. The specific characteristics create the personality trait. Circle the feelings you experience frequently and intensely. Repeat this process with the personality traits.

EMOTIONAL VOCABULARY

PRIMARY FEELING STATES:

Angry

aggressive
agitated
annoyed
bitter
burned out
critical
disgusted
disregarded
disrespected
enraged

envious
fed up
frustrated
furious
hostile
ignored
impatient
irate
irritated
livid

mad
outraged
perturbed
resentful
seething
ticked off
unappreciated
violent
worked up

Confused

anxious
awkward
baffled
bewildered
bothered
crazy
dazed
disorganized
disorientated
distracted
disturbed
embarrassed

frustrated
helpless
hopeless
humiliated
lost
mixed up
panicky
paralyzed
perplexed
puzzled
shocked
stuck

stunned
surprised
tangled
trapped
troubled
uncertain
uncomfortable
undecided
unsure
upset
weak

Fearful

afraid	insecure	tense
anxious	intimidated	terrified
apprehensive	jumpy	threatened
cautious	lonely	uneasy
crazy	nervous	unsafe
edgy	panicky	unsure
frightened	paralyzed	worried
horrified	shaky	

Happy

alive	fulfilled	refreshed
amused	glad	relaxed
calm	good	relieved
cheerful	great	satisfied
content	hopeful	spirited
delighted	humorous	thankful
ecstatic	loving	thrilled
elated	nurturing	up
energized	overjoyed	validated
excited	peaceful	warm
fortunate	pleased	wonderful
friendly	proud	

Sad

awful	disturbed	low
bad	down	miserable
blue	embarrassed	painful
bummed out	gloomy	sorry
crushed	glum	terrible

depressed
desperate
devastated
disappointed
dissatisfied

hateful
hopeless
hurt
lonely
lost

uneasy
unhappy
unloved
upset

Strong

active
alert
angry
assertive
bold
brave
capable
confident
determined

eager
energetic
happy
healthy
honest
intelligent
intense
loving

positive
powerful
resilient
secure
self-assured
sure
survivor
tough

Weak

abused
ashamed
defenseless
demoralized
discouraged
disorganized
disrespected
embarrassed
exhausted
fragile
frustrate

guilty
helpless
horrible
ill
inadequate
incapable
insecure
intimidated
overwhelmed
passive
powerless

procrastinate
run-down
shaky
shy
sick
stressed
stupid
tired
unsure
useless
worthless

Personalize:

List your primary feeling states:

_____

_____

_____

_____

PERSONALITY TRAITS

<u>Accepting</u>

discerning	peaceful	sensible
non-judgmental	rational	tolerant
objective	self-aware	wise
open-minded		

<u>Calm</u>

peaceful	self-possessed	stable
quiet	serene	still

<u>Creative</u>

artistic	individualistic	romantic
dramatic	imaginative	sentimental
expressive	inventive	witty

Effective/responsible

assertive	dedicated	motivating
capable	dependable	organized
careful	diplomatic	persevering
committed	disciplined	practical
competent	ethical	principled
confident	focused	productive
conscientious	hard-working	reliable
co-operative	honest	resourceful
decisive	industrious	strong

Judgemental

critical	perfectionist	uncompromising
inflexible	rigid	unsympathetic
intolerant		

Loving

affectionate	generous	selfless
appreciative	helpful	sincere
attentive	kind	sympathetic
caring	merciful	tender
comforting	nurturing	thoughtful
compassionate	patient	trustworthy
empathetic	protective	warm
forgiving		

Manipulative

appeasing	discouraging	needy
blaming	enabling	resentful

bitter
controlling
dependent

guilt-instilling
insincere

self-pitying
suppressive

Rageful/dominating

accusatory
antagonistic
bad-tempered
brooding
coercive
confrontational
contemptuous
controlling
cruel
defiant
demanding

destructive
dictatorial
impatient
malicious
mean
oppressive
over-bearing
patronizing
petty
possessive
predatory

rejecting
remorseless
resentful
ruthless
stubborn
sulking
unaware
unsympathetic
vengeful
violent

Self - Absorbed

boastful
conceited
demanding
dismissive

envious
petty
petulant
presumptuous

pretentious
self-indulgent
selfish

Withdrawn

apathetic
anti-social
brooding
complacent
confused
despondent

indifferent
melancholy
moody
phobic
pre-occupied
reclusive

resistant
secretive
self-doubting
unreflective
unresponsive
vulnerable

Personalize:

List your dominant personality traits:

DESTINATION

As with all journeys there is a destination. The destination of the healing process is one of discovery. Discover your true self by breaking free of the lies of abuse.

Personalize:

Take a few minutes right now to write down a description of the kind of person you would like to be. Use your lists to help you.

_____

_____

_____

_____

_____

_____

_____

_____

It is my belief the person you want to be, is in fact, the person you *already* are.

The person who has been hidden beneath all the lies and confusion created by the abuse in your life. Our dominant feeling states influence how our personality traits are demonstrated in a powerful way. Positive feeling states bring out our positive personality traits. For instance, it's not uncommon for a person who habitually feels **weak**: ashamed, defenseless, insecure, and worthless to act their feeling state through the **manipulative trait**: appeasing, enabling, needy, insincere, self-pitying. Thus the manipulation trait may become one of the person's dominant traits which they use consistently in their interactions with others. In contrast a person who typically feels **strong**: assertive, capable, confident, secure, self-assured, will act out their feeling through personality traits such as **effective/responsible,** calm and accepting. Each of us possesses strengths and weaknesses in our character or personality, what we would say are the *good* and the *bad* aspects of ourselves. None of us were created to be better or worse than anyone else.

Fear:

"I didn't realize how often I show my feelings through the manipulative trait. One of my most common feeling states is fear. I'm so worried that people won't like me or be disappointed in me that I am constantly trying to appease everyone. I always thought of myself as an honest person but I now realize how often I'm insincere. I don't tell people what I really think because I'm afraid of how they might react if they don't like what I have to say. I seldom say no to my children because I'm afraid they wouldn't love me anymore. I'm teaching them they never have to take responsibility for themselves by spoiling them and never giving them consequences for bad behavior."

Weak:

"People would be really surprised if they knew how powerless I feel a lot of the time. I feel guilty unless everything is going well for everybody. I feel like I'm responsible for other people's feelings and actions. I end up feeling overwhelmed. I sometimes show these feelings through the Rageful/Dominating trait. I resent feeling so responsible. I know I can get petty and impatient about the little things. I don't want people to know how weak and needy I really feel. I'm afraid I'll be taken advantage of. I try to make sure everyone knows I'm in control that way they won't try to control me. All my relationships seem to be one struggle after another.

Strong:

"Right now in my life I feel strong. I always have more energy when I feel like this. I believe in myself. I know I have the capability and determination to accomplish my goals and solve whatever problems arise. I find it easier to be assertive with people. In reviewing the vocabulary lists I realize these positive feelings show through the traits of calm, effective/responsible and accepting. When I accept myself situations and people don't threaten me because I know no matter what happens I can trust myself to do what is right for me.

Personalize:

Write down the personality traits that are commonly demonstrated through your feeling states.

_____

_____

_____

_____

_____

_____

_____

ACCEPTING YOU HAVE BEEN ABUSED

To move forward in your healing process there are several things you must do. First and foremost you must acknowledge and accept the abuse has occurred.

"You will continue to live in a world of pain if you refuse to admit what you are really suffering from."

- Oprah Winfrey

Accepting that you have been abused does not mean condoning or excusing it. It simply means you acknowledge that it happened and it caused you harm.

No matter what the circumstances surrounding the abuse you need to understand and accept that it was not your fault. Regardless of what you may have been told or what you came to believe, there is nothing you did, nothing you said, nothing about your appearance that *made* another human being violate you.

All forms of abuse are a misuse of power.

Physical and emotional abuse cannot be justified by labeling it discipline. The purpose of discipline is to *build up* not to *tear down* the child. Authentic discipline supports the child in developing respect, self-control, boundaries, competency, responsibility and empathy. Discipline does not leave the child confused, humiliated, shamed and angry. Discipline does not wound the child's body, mind and spirit. When the child is wounded abuse has occurred.

"When we were kids my mother would hit us and humiliate us if we did something she didn't like, which was most of the time. She never let you explain anything; if you tried you got a slap in the face for talking back. The teachers always said I was a nice well-mannered child. I really was just frightened. My brother was forever getting in trouble at school, talking back and fighting. He would get it at school and then twice as bad when he got home. My mother would beat him black and blue. She said if it was the last thing she ever did she would teach him to behave. She was so furious at him for 'embarrassing' her and making her 'look bad' that she would be practically foaming at the

mouth. The more she beat him the worse he got and the quieter I got. Getting into trouble was the one way my brother had of getting even with her. I secretly admired him."

"I had a teacher who, when you got a low mark, would read it out to the class and make jokes about what you might have been doing instead of studying. I wasn't a very good student so this happened to me a lot. I remember once studying really hard for a test and getting a good mark. The teacher asked me in front of the class if I had cheated because he didn't think I was smart enough to have done that well. To this day I feel sick with embarrassment when I think of it. I learned the safest place to be is in the middle; don't attract attention to yourself one way or another"

In the case of sexual abuse there are two scenarios in particular in which victims have great difficulty accepting that what has occurred is abusive.

In situations where sexual abuse is not violent or physically painful the victim may experience pleasurable physical sensations. For many survivors this develops into the belief that if they experienced pleasure they must have wanted it to happen. This is simply not true. It only means the body responded to sexual stimulation in the way it was designed to.

In cases that involve long term abuse, particularly if it began at an early age, victims may initiate sexual contact with the perpetrator or they may simply have stopped trying to avoid or resist him/her. Children who have been introduced to sexuality or *sexualized* in this way are often so confused in relation to love and normal sexual behavior they will often initiate sexual contact as a means of meeting their natural non-sexual needs for love, safety and acceptance. This doesn't mean the victim has been a willing participant. Nothing could be further from the truth. It is however a clear indication of the serious degree of distortion and trauma being experienced by the victim.

Abuse is an act of corrupted will; the offender's not the victim's.

"No one knows what it is like to feel like this. I know I deserve it and I can't forget that. When I told my mom she said it was my fault. She said I must have done something to make my brother act like that. I know that must be true because I hated it but I liked it too."

"I can sometimes understand what people mean when they tell me what happened when I was a kid was not my fault. But whose fault was it when I got older? I'm the one who drank until I didn't care who I had sex with."

"When I was twelve my friend's dad started fooling around with me. I knew it was wrong but it felt good to be someone 'special.' He said he couldn't stand to be near me without touching me. At home no one even noticed whether I was there. He told me he loved me and wanted to be my boyfriend."

To know you have been abused and keep it inside yourself is not easy, but to speak it out loud or put it in writing is not only incredibly difficult but very painful. Acknowledging the abuse outside of you makes it *real*. It is a powerful step in breaking down the coping strategies that at one time protected you from the pain but are now barriers to healing. It also ends the *secrets* you have kept at great emotional cost. If this is the first time you have acknowledged the abuse outside yourself it will be painful and frightening. Don't loose heart, remember these are the *feelings of the child* you once were. You are no longer that powerless child. You are an adult who is strong. You are a survivor.

"I am a victim of abuse. I was emotionally and sexually abused as a child and physically abused as an adult. Of all the abuse in my life the emotional abuse/neglect was the worst because it wasn't recognized as abuse. I just didn't exist as a person. I was of no particular importance or use. I was only seen when I was in need of correction. It hurts so much to acknowledge how little I meant. I know some of the choices I made in my life would have been different if I had understood I had value. Even as I write this it seems false like I'm making excuses for myself. I feel guilty, like I'm being disloyal and just feeling sorry for myself. Most of my feelings are of not being a real person, not belonging and not feeling worthy. I feel like I'm different from everybody else in my family, weak, incompetent, an 'air head.' I feel angry and afraid much of the time. I can't say at who. I can feel myself pushing people away, but I can't seem to stop it. It's hard for me to understand why people care about me, why they want to help me. I don't even like myself.........."

Personalize:

Using your word lists to help you write a statement that acknowledges the abuse in your life. As in the example above include how you are feeling right now, emotionally and physically.

Take a few minutes and just be aware of what you are feeling right now. Don't try to deny, change or explain them. Feelings are not right or wrong, they are just what they are. You can pretend you don't feel the way you do but pretending or denying doesn't change or erase your true feelings. You are the owner of your feelings, they belong to you, they are real, they are valid and they are to be respected. Remember you can feel the feeling without acting it out through a negative personality trait. Choose to demonstrate your feelings through your positive traits. You can choose to be accepting of your feelings; you can choose to be loving, compassionate, merciful and nurturing toward your self.

How difficult was it for you not to blame yourself or make excuses for your abuser? If you had difficulties take a few minutes to answer the following questions

As a child what kind of power did I possess over my abuser(s) that enabled me to force them to abuse me?

_____

_____

_____

_____

Are there any circumstances under which I believe it is acceptable to abuse a child?

_____

_____

_____

_____

_____

_____

Am I afraid to be angry at the person(s) that abused me? If so, why?

_____

_____

_____

_____

_____

_____

Why do some people abuse?

Every person who has ever been abused has asked why. Even when the victim has not yet fully acknowledged that abuse has occurred they will still ask the question in some form. *Why aren't I good enough? What am I doing wrong?* In truth there will never be a satisfactory answer for this question. The very act of asking why implies that if one searches long enough they will find an acceptable reason. There isn't an acceptable reason.

As adults we understand there are certain circumstances which can increase a person's susceptibility to commit abuse. Often abusers were abused themselves as children and continue to struggle with unresolved feelings of rage and insecurity, or perhaps they are struggling to cope with an addiction or stress. Whatever the situation may be the abuser's susceptibility is not an excuse or a reason to abuse. You have been abused and it was wrong. Healing doesn't require you to hate your abuser(s) in fact you may love them and wish to forgive them. The more you love those who have offended against you the greater the chance is you will try to excuse their behavior. Finding excuses for the wrongs committed against you will not lead to true forgiveness. In fact making excuses will lead away from forgiveness. *To truly forgive one must first understand and acknowledge what it is you are forgiving.* You may have very conflicted feelings especially when your abuser is someone you love. There is no *right* way to feel about the person who abused you. There is no *right* way to handle the relationship. There is only *your* way. There is only one rule; you cannot allow yourself to be further abused. You don't have to stop loving your abuser before you can admit you were hurt by the abuse. By the same token you don't have to love someone who abused you because they are related to you or you believe you *should* love them. Perhaps you will decide that you love and forgive your abuser but choose not to have them in your life because their presence is damaging to you. You can confront your abuser or not, you can stay in relationship with them or not. The choices are *yours*. What you can't do however is to continue to deny or distort your feelings. Remember the road to healing is *truth*.

The truth is no one has the power to make another person abuse them. The truth is there is never a circumstance when it is acceptable to abuse another. The truth is you have a right to the feelings you have about being abused and the feelings you have about your abuser. The truth is abusing another person is a choice and regardless of how a person may have been conditioned by their own experiences they are still accountable for their actions. Don't be afraid to move forward in your healing process.

The truth will set you free.

IDENTIFY CORE BELIEFS

Making the connection between how you were impacted by the abuse and how it is influencing you in the present is also a necessary step in the healing process.

The first step in making these connections is to identify what your *core belief* is. Broken down into its simplest terms you operate from a belief system that says, ***"I am good" or "I am bad"***

Everything in your life is filtered through your core belief.

Your feelings are influenced by the beliefs you hold about yourself. When you value yourself, "I am good" you will consciously draw on your positive traits, acting on your negative feelings states in a manner that cares for and protects the self, thereby changing the negative state to a positive one. When you don't value yourself, "I am bad" your negative feeling states will be acted out through your negative traits in destructive ways that don't care for or protect the self but rather reinforce and escalate the negative feeling state.

Personalize:

To identify your core belief; first determine whether your frequent feelings are positive or negative. Use your emotional vocabulary ratings to help you. You may find it helpful to categorize these by environment: home, work and social.

EXAMPLE:

My most frequently experienced feelings are:

Home:	**Work:**	**Social:**
rejected	*capable*	*inadequate*
inadequate	*frustrated*	*fearful*
sad		*rejected*
frustrated		

As you review your list of feelings think about how you act upon them and which core belief do they support?

Home

"My feeling state at home is most often negative. It seems like what I want is of no importance or at least not as important as what my partner wants. It doesn't seem to matter how often I say something I get ignored. I usually act on it by withdrawing and then by yelling. Nothing changes and I only feel worse."

Work

"At work I feel capable but I'm also frustrated because I don't get the recognition I deserve for how hard I work. I haven't done anything about it though; I just keep my mouth shut and hope I'll get noticed. I am really angry with myself for never saying anything."

Social

"I don't go out much and when I do I usually end up worrying that I said or did something to offend someone. I feel fearful and inadequate. I act by avoiding social situations. When an occasion comes up that's unavoidable I sometimes drink too much and then later regret it.

My most frequently experienced feeling states are:

_____

_____

_____

_____

I act upon them by:

_____

_____

_____

_____

_____

_____

My feeling states support the core belief by:

_____

_____

_____

_____

_____

_____

IDENTIFY SYMPTOMS OF ABUSE

From your core belief and the subsequent symptoms that develop, a secondary system is formed. Your secondary beliefs reflect and reinforce your core belief. Case in point, if you believe that you are essentially bad, it is likely you have come to believe that you are unworthy, incompetent, undeserving and so on. You become trapped in a vicious circle of damaging thoughts, feelings and actions. These are the symptoms of abuse.

The symptoms of abuse can be divided into two broad categories, *internal* and *external*. Internal symptoms are manifest in what you feel and think external symptoms in what you do. Symptoms are as diverse as the victims themselves. They are a product of the degree of trauma, individual personality traits, learned behaviors and other life experiences and influences. Some individuals demonstrate strong external symptoms such as addictions, aggression and panic attacks while others may exhibit external symptoms which are barely detectable. However, there is one area where all victims are inevitably impacted and that is within the context of their relationships.

A person who is operating from a belief system that they are *bad* will have little or no expectation their emotional needs will be responded to unless some form of manipulation or coercion is used. For example a woman may choose to suppress her own emotional needs and seek only to satisfy the needs of others. She does this in the hope of winning the love and acceptance of others. A man believes that to keep his wife attached to him he must control every aspect of her life. Although their behavior is different it is motivated by the same need; to be loved and to be accepted. Regardless of the external methods used the victim feels isolated and uncared for, disconnected from others. In my work as an abuse counselor I have heard people describe their lives as having an *unreal* quality. I get a mental picture of the person standing behind a pane of glass. They can observe others enjoying the warmth of companionship, they can imitate what they see but still somehow they remain apart. They *act* their lives, playing their roles and waiting to see how the audience will respond. Directed always by the response of others, watching for clues that tell them who they are and if they are good enough. Abuse victims learn, by necessity, to be proficient actors. Often becoming so immersed in their roles they do not know what their own truths are. Abuse places a barrier between the victim and their *true self*.

"Will I ever be a real person? Will there be a place for me?"

"Things that happened in my past, the things I lost make me feel I can never live a normal life."

"If you knew what really happened, what I did, you wouldn't bother with me. I try to be what people want me to be, that way they will never know how bad I really am."

"I end up driving away the people I love. My husband says I smother him. I don't understand all I'm trying to do is look after him. He will leave if he doesn't need me."

To assist you in understanding how you have been impacted by the abuse in your life I have included a list of common symptoms. These have been loosely categorized by age. The frequency and severity of the symptom is usually a good indicator of the degree of trauma experienced. Check the symptoms you have experienced. Add any that may not have been included on the lists.

YOUNG CHILDREN
- Regression (acts younger than age)
- Aggressive destructive behavior
- Inappropriate knowledge of and excessive interest in sex
- Inappropriate touching
- Hyperactivity/disruptive behavior
- Fearful/timid (generalized or specific fears)
- Withdrawn (doesn't participate in usual activities or relationships)
- Lacks concentration
- Depression/disrupted eating and sleeping habits
- Nightmares
- Bedwetting
- Stomach aches/ head aches
- Emotionally upset (cries easily, overly sensitive)
- Gives or receives affection indiscriminately
- Speech disorders
- Demonstrates emotional detachment
- Negative self-statements
- Emotionally unresponsive or numb

ADOLESCENTS
- Abusive to others and/or self
- Drug/alcohol abuse
- Eating disorders
- Problems in school (friends, grades, truancy)
- Delinquency (lying, stealing)
- Running away
- Sexual acting out

- Age inappropriate dating
- Taking risks
- Low self-esteem
- Suicidal thoughts and attempts
- Self-mutilation
- Depression
- Overly compliant (tries too hard to please others)
- Passive resistant
- Withdrawn
- Pseudo-mature
- Overly responsible
- Idealizing family

ADULTS

Damage to Self-Esteem and Self-Image
- Feelings of worthlessness
- Feeling in the way or left out
- Chronic feelings of guilt or shame
- Tendency to blame self for whatever goes wrong
- Tendency to blame others for whatever goes wrong
- Inability to complete tasks
- Tendency to sabotage success
- Tendency to be victimized by others

Relationship Problems
- Difficulty trusting others
- Being distant and aloof
- Tendency to be involved with destructive, abusive people
- Lack of empathy or concern for others
- Deep sense of isolation
- Difficulty with physical affection
- Secretive/evasive/tendency to withhold information
- Tendency to give yourself away
- Difficulty with authority figures
- Difficulty communicating desires, thoughts and feelings
- Difficulty receiving from others
- Sexual problems

Emotional Problems
- Intense feelings of anger and rage that sometimes erupt
- Mood swings
- Chronic depression
- Dissociation
- Extreme fears and phobias
- Sleep disturbances
- Addictions
- Obsessive/compulsive behavior
- Eating disorders
- Flashbacks or hallucinations
- Abusive behavior toward others or self

Physical Problems
- Somatic problems (aches, pains, chronic illness)

Personalize:

It is important to understand how the symptoms you experienced and how others responded to them has influenced the perception you have of yourself. As a result of the symptoms a *secondary belief* system developed. This system reinforced the core belief, *"I am bad"* and determined, to a large extent, how you began to think, feel and then function in the world.

Write down the symptoms you checked off. Categorize them by age and then write down how others responded and the feelings you had as a result. You may want to use your Emotional Vocabulary List to help you. I have also included an example to help you.

Young Child

Symptom	Other's Response	My Feelings
bedwetting	anger	ashamed
	ridicule	anxious
		worried
		embarrassed
		humiliated
emotionally upset	impatient	afraid
	teased	isolated

Young Child:

_____

_____

_____

_____

_____

Adolescent:

_____

_____

_____

_____

_____

Adult:

_____

_____

_____

_____

_____

_____

_____

Now go back and beside each of the feelings you have listed write the *primary* feeling category it appears under on the Emotional Vocabulary List. These primary feeling states determined the secondary beliefs that developed in your life. Each time you experienced a particular feeling the more *fixed* the secondary belief became in your life. Use the following example as a guideline.

Feeling	**Secondary Belief**
Ashamed	WEAK
Anxious	FEARFUL
Worried	FEARFUL
Embarrassed	WEAK
Humiliated	CONFUSED/WEAK

From the abuse symptoms came the feelings and resulting beliefs that have dominated your life. Symptoms by which you have defined yourself as a person. This is not who you are. This false identity is the poison fruit of abuse.

IDENTIFY DISTORTED THINKING

Distorted thinking is a direct result of the flawed beliefs you carry about yourself. These secondary beliefs were shaped as a result of the symptoms of your abuse. Like many of you I have a computer that I use mainly for work related tasks. I am competent at using the features designed to do these tasks. In fact I have become so familiar with the daily operations I don't really need to think very much about what I am doing. I just automatically push the right buttons. However I am not nearly so proficient at using the fun features. I seldom use them and so they remain unfamiliar and somewhat mystifying to me. Our thinking process can be likened to using a computer. We function according to what has been programmed into us. These are the programs or the thinking patterns which are so familiar to us we just automatically go through the operations. We input the information and press enter. All incoming information is then filtered, or processed if you will, through our belief system.

This process begins with the belief or perception we have of ourselves. Next comes the feeling or thought, (your feelings affect your thoughts > your thoughts affect your feelings) and then the resulting behavior.

How can you accurately identify what is wrong in your life or effectively manage the feelings that sometimes threaten to overwhelm you when your belief system is based on a lie. The truth is you cannot. To make sense of it you attach your thoughts, feelings and subsequent behavior on what is happening in the present. Imagine a long hall way with rooms on either side. The door to each room is labeled with a feeling. Inside each of these rooms are stored all the unresolved feelings which occurred as a result of the abuse you suffered. Each time you experience one of those feelings in the present the door gets opened and all the feeling pushed behind the door come pouring out. For example if all the rage you felt as a child had to be denied so you could survive you may find yourself enraged over situations in the present that realistically should produce only moderate anger. Or perhaps you have been so afraid of losing control that you will not allow yourself to express any anger at all and continue to push all your anger behind the door. In either situation the end result will be the same, a normal healthy feeling is distorted and expressed in an unhealthy way. Feelings may be turned outward in an excessive display of emotion, or inward, rigidly suppressing the feeling in an attempt to deny its existence. When your feelings are not honestly acknowledged and processed, solving problems is impossible. How can anyone resolve relationship issues which stem from chronic unresolved anger when the true source of the anger is denied or believed to come from outside the self? How can you get the right answer to the problem when you have the wrong equation?

An emotional equation looks like this:

belief > thought > feeling > action

EXAMPLE:

A toddler demands a toy when shopping with his parent. The parent responds by telling the child no. The toddler has a temper tantrum and attracts the attention of other shoppers.

Unhealthy Equation: Core Belief "I am bad"

I am powerless > I don't know what to do > overwhelmed > gives in to the child

   (belief)   (thought)   (feeling)   (action)

The child learns that he can control his parent and get what he wants by screaming. The child learns to disrespect his parent.

Healthy Equation: Core Belief "I am good"

I have power > I am in control > confident > calmly removes the child

   (belief)   (thought)   (feeling)   (action)

The child learns that his parent is in control and there are consequences for his actions. The child learns to respect his parent.

Whatever action you take reinforces your belief. In the unhealthy equation the parent's action resulted in increased feelings of powerlessness. In the healthy equation the parent's actions increase feelings of personal power.

EXAMPLE:

Susan goes shopping with her friend Jane. Jane suggests they go out for supper after shopping. Susan phones home to tell her husband she will be home later than she expected because of the change in plans. Even though they had no plans Don, her husband, is angry and accuses Susan of not wanting to spend time with him.

Core Belief: "I am bad"

Secondary Belief: Weak, Fearful

Feeling: Embarrassed, Guilty

Thought: I must have done something wrong.

Action: Makes an excuse and goes home. Spends the evening placating Don.

Core Belief: "I am good"

Secondary Belief: Strong

Feeling: Irritated

Thought: He is being unreasonable.

Action: Has supper with Jane and enjoys herself. Susan refuses to take responsibility for Don's childish behavior.

Personalize:

In what ways do the beliefs you carry about yourself influence your life?

Write down any stressful situations that occur repeatedly in your life and then analyze them. Sometimes it is easier to work backwards, starting with the action, then thoughts and feelings, then the secondary and core belief. You may find it beneficial to categorize these as you did with the primary feeling states: home, work, and social.

Identify Distorted Thinking

Personalize:

How many of the destructive beliefs you developed as a child are the same ones which are influencing your thoughts, feelings and actions today? Write down your early memories, try to do at least three. Look at the content of these carefully. What are the feelings you experienced in each of these memories? Is there a theme which emerges?

Remember these beliefs are the byproduct of the symptoms of your abuse.

"After writing down my earliest memories I realized most involved being verbally abused. I grew up feeling ashamed of myself for being such a 'hopeless case', who could never do anything right. I realize that I have never gotten over that feeling. I'm always worried that I said or did something wrong. I just know I'm going to make a mistake or disappoint people in some way. I am so sick of feeling guilty and ashamed I get really pissed off at people and end up being verbally abusive."

The theme that emerges for me is: *What's the use of trying? I'll just screw it up anyway so I might as well get them before they get me.*

My memories are:

_____

_____

_____

_____

_____

_____

IDENTIFY COPING STRATEGIES

The purpose of coping strategies is to protect you from emotional pain. Minimizing and forgetting are the most common strategies used, particularly by children, to survive abuse. *"If I don't think about it I won't feel it."* Coping in this manner was likely necessary for the child to psychologically survive but when carried into adulthood it becomes a hindrance to achieving a healthy emotional life. The coping strategies you use don't remain exclusive to the abusive incidents. If you learned as a child to cope with your feelings by avoidance you will likely cope in the same way when similar feelings are triggered in the present day.

No matter how skilled you become at avoiding the pain and fear it remains perfectly preserved within you. Like ancient hieroglyphics, gouged into the wall of a cave, still present but lost to the light of awareness. Unrecognized perhaps, but still carried forward into every aspect of your life. Unacknowledged your pain masquerades as something else, lack of control, rigid control, bad relationships, eating disorders, chronic illness, phobias, compulsions, obsessions, addiction and the list goes on. Survivors struggle in their daily lives to cope with the symptoms of their abuse. No matter what coping strategies are employed they all have the same function, to protect the victim from the pain of facing the *badness* they believe is at the core of their being.

As different as symptoms and coping strategies may be; abuse victims all have one thing in common, they are desperately trying to create a place of emotional safety. A place where they have some sense of power and control. For the victim there was no control, no personal power. They were at the mercy of the abuser. An emotionally healthy adult balances their own need for power and control with respect and understanding that others have the same need, thereby establishing relationships based on mutual empathy and support. In contrast an emotionally unhealthy adult will attempt to avoid feelings of powerlessness either by dominating and controlling another person and/or environment, or by simply relinquishing control of their lives to someone or something else.

If, for instance, you are by nature and circumstance a perfectionist you may seek to gain a sense of power and control through your external environment. You focus your efforts on organizing your life in attempt to achieve perfection. This can apply to all aspects of your life or only a selected few. You operate on the belief '*When my world is perfect I will be safe from the badness that is me, or at least my inadequacies will be well hidden. My perfection will prove that I am worthy.*' To attain this goal you become critical of yourself and sometimes of others. If your faulty belief system tells you that you are inadequate or inferior any present circumstance that produces those feelings will feel unbearable to you. It is viewed as confirmation that indeed you are a "bad" person. You may immediately assume you must have done something wrong or you may become defensive and angry refusing to acknowledge anything you perceive as criticism. In either situation the motivation is the same; you are trying to protect yourself from the pain and fear which has plagued you throughout your life. You may, in your struggle for safety determine there is no room for error in your life, no room for mistakes. You fail to make the connection that the intensity of your feelings stem from the past not the present. In reality perfection is an unattainable goal, not because you are deficient in some way but simply because it is not humanly possible to be perfect. But it is not reality that drives you; it is *fear*. Fear of being unwanted, worthless, abandoned, controlled, condemned, harmed, deprived and so on.

The truth is; *the degree to which you are driven to be in control or the degree to which you relinquish control is a good indication of how out of control and powerless you truly are.*

In situations where your personality functions from a secondary belief system that says you are powerless, you may feel incapable of creating a place of safety for yourself. You believe you have no way of impacting yourself, others or your environment in a positive way. You try to gain a sense of safety by allowing someone or something else to take charge of your life.

'If someone more capable…stronger…smarter…is in charge I will be safe.'

'If I try to be what others want me to be I will be safe.'

'If I drink… work…play…hard enough and don't think, I will be safe.'

The more extreme your emotional distress is the more extreme your coping strategies become. You attempt to distance yourself from the pain and fear in whatever way best suits your natural personality type and what is available to you. Within you remain all the distortions and faulty beliefs. You seldom, if ever, make the connection between these and your abusive experiences. The belief *I am bad* is so deeply ingrained in your psyche it doesn't even occur to you to challenge it.

As an abused child you had no way of protecting yourself or keeping yourself safe. You began to filter all information through:

I am bad > your symptoms > secondary beliefs

You had to find a way to cope with the *bad* person who lived inside you. The only way to survive was to find someway to contain the emotional and psychological pain. Typically the coping strategies or defenses that allowed you to survive as a child become self-defeating in adulthood. As you grew older it became necessary to construct additional defenses to contain the unhealthy perceptions you developed about yourself and the world around you. In reality your coping strategies are no longer protecting you but in fact, by keeping the truth hidden, have become symptoms in and of themselves. If for instance you have used escaping as a primary coping strategy you may have developed an addiction which in turn is symptomatic of your abuse. In this manner your coping strategies may be depriving you from experiencing healthy, satisfying relationships with yourself, others and even your environments.

Personalize:

The following list has been included to help you identify the coping strategies you use on a frequent basis. Answer the questions using the categories of:

N - Never   S - Sometimes   O - Often

Remember the frequency and degree to which you use these strategies is indicative of the severity of trauma you experienced.

Dissociation:

Dissociation is an altered state of consciousness with the sole purpose of separating the victim from the feelings associated with the trauma.

Do you:

_____ have no awareness or memory of what is happening around you?

_____ frequently daydream?

_____ think or talk about your abuse with little or no feeling?

_____ lack concentration?

_____ have trouble remembering things past and present?

Controlling:

All adult survivors of abuse have, to some degree, a problem with control. They either attempt to excessively control everything in their life or surrender too much of their control to others. In either case you do not have a true sense of your own power.

Do you:

_____ strive to be perfect?

_____ expect others to strive for perfection?

_____ feel satisfied with yourself and/or others?

_____ always have a plan?

_____ need to keep busy all the time?

_____ use guilt and/or flattery to get what you want/need from others?

_____ believe there is only one right way to think, feel or do things?

_____ try to force others to see things your way?

_____ say "I should" or "you should" frequently?

_____ keep your feelings to yourself?

_____ try to be everything to everybody?

_____ take time for yourself?

_____ have certain rituals that you perform repeatedly?

_____ have unhealthy eating habits?

_____ obsess about your appearance?

_____ obsess about your environment and possessions?

Escaping:

Escaping is one of the most common coping strategies used by adolescents and young adults.

Do you or have you in the past:

_____ spend an excessive amount of time on a specific activity, such as work or a hobby as a means of avoiding feeling?

_____ run away?

_____ thought about suicide?

_____ attempted suicide?

_____ physically hurt yourself intentionally?

_____ struggle with addiction? (drugs, alcohol, gambling, sex, food, shopping)

_____ have problems with shoplifting or other unlawful behaviors?

Forgetting:

This is the most common coping strategy used by young children. All 'brain' memory is forgotten and only 'body and feeling' memory remain.

Do you:

_____ have significant gaps in your childhood memories?

_____ experience sensations or emotions that you don't understand?

Minimizing:

When we cope in this manner we down play the impact the abuse has on us.

Do you:

_____ tell yourself that what happened was 'not really that bad'

_____ find yourself minimizing other people's feelings believing they are over-reacting and being too emotional or unreasonable?

Rationalizing:

Rationalizing occurs when we attempt to explain the abuse away or make excuses for it.

Do you:

_____ find a reason or explanation for why the abuse happened?

_____ even though you may not agree with the way you were treated you still try to convince yourself and others that there was a purpose for the abuse

"My dad used his fists on us but at least we learned respect."

Guilt:

This is, in my opinion, the most commonplace coping strategy. Typically abuse victims experience excessive feelings of guilt. Feeling guilty in an odd way allows victims to maintain some sense of control. Guilt implies that the victim had enough control to have done things differently, to have made a choice that would have changed the outcome. In addition guilt keeps the victim focused on improving, being better, stronger, smarter…, and away from the pain of being abused. Guilt is particularly prevalent when the abuser was someone who was loved by the victim.

Do you:

_____ blame yourself when you encounter a problem?

_____ call yourself names or make derogatory self-statements?

_____ allow others to disrespect you?

_____ worry excessively about what you say or do?

_____ assume you have done something wrong if someone appears to be upset?

_____ constantly apologize?

_____ feel responsible for the emotional well-being of everyone?

Physiological Defenses:

When physiological defenses are engaged the pain of the abuse is experienced through the body. This type of defense allows the victim to focus on the pain in the body and away from the emotional pain. The body gives voice to the pain which the victim will not allow their mind and heart to express.

Do you:

_____ frequently have headaches, stomach problems or other reoccurring ailments?

_____ make frequent visits to the doctor?

_____ have difficulty having ailments diagnosed?

Sexualized Behavior:

This coping strategy is most common with victims of sexual abuse. It is not unusual for survivors to try and meet non-sexual needs through sexualized behavior. Sexual promiscuity and submissiveness often becomes the means used by the victim to try and gain love, approval, safety and security.

Do you:

_____ have numerous sexual partners?

_____ have sex with people you don't know well?

_____ have sex when you don't want to?

_____ dress provocatively to attract attention?

Personalize:

As a child you were unable to challenge the lies you were told by your abusers, or deal with the overwhelming feelings that resulted. You went into *survival mode* putting up defense strategies which many of you are still using. You remain strongly influenced by your childhood fears. If you remain unaware of what your true fears are and where they originated from you cannot hope to conquer them. Examine your personal lists of symptoms and secondary beliefs to help you pinpoint what your basic fears are.

Determine the frequency and intensity of your fears by rating them.

N - Never   S - Sometimes   O - Often

Common Fears:

_____ fear of being unloved

_____ fear of being unworthy

_____ fear of being unwanted

_____ fear of having no identity of your own

_____ fear of being powerless

_____ fear of being controlled

_____ fear of being incompetent

_____ fear of having no significance or importance

_____ fear of being rejected

_____ fear of being abandoned

_____ fear of being in pain

_____ fear of being deprived

_____ fear of being harmed

_____ fear of being alone

_____ fear of being humiliated

How do your fears and coping strategies work together?

EXAMPLE:

Fear: Being Controlled/Being Powerless **Coping Strategy:** Controlling

"When I feel like I am not in full control of what is going on in my life I get really possessed with my relationships and my environment. Everyone and everything has to be perfect."

_____

_____

_____

_____

_____

_____

What coping strategies did you use as a child?

_____

_____

_____

_____

_____

_____

What did these strategies protect you from?

_____

_____

_____

_____

_____

How did those strategies harm or hinder you?

_____

_____

_____

_____

_____

What coping strategies do you use as an adult?

_____

_____

_____

_____

_____

What do these coping strategies protect you from?

_____

_____

_____

_____

_____

How do these coping strategies harm or hinder you?

_____

_____

_____

_____

_____

_____

What coping strategies have you carried from childhood into adulthood?

_____

_____

_____

_____

_____

_____

How do these coping strategies help or hinder you now?

_____

_____

_____

_____

_____

_____

INTEGRATION

Another key task of the healing process is integration. The victim must integrate the abusive experiences into themselves.

How can you be emotionally and psychologically wounded and function as though you were not? It would be like breaking your fingers and still expecting your hand to perform with precision. When this isn't possible you berate yourself and wonder what is wrong with you when you fail to do what seems to come so easily to others. Unfortunately *forgetting* not *healing* is often encouraged as the best method for dealing with abuse trauma. The victim, the people who love them and sometimes even the professionals the victim goes to for help may believe forgetting is the best choice. Encouraging you to forget might be intended to be helpful but in fact it is not.

Most abuse victims have heard or said things like:

"You can't change what happened in the past so just forget about it."

"It doesn't really bother me, it happened a long time ago."

"What good does it do to think about all that stuff? It just makes me feel bad."

"I've been told I'm feeling sorry for myself and I guess I am."

"My family doctor told the best thing I can do for myself is get a hobby, something that would take my mind off myself."

Why can't you leave it in the past? To an abuse victim this question is often perceived as an accusation. It implies that there is a weakness in the survivor and a strong person would be able to 'get on with it.' It is true you need to find a way to move forward but the only *real* way to do that is to stop trying to run from your pain and face it. Supportive responses are those which validate the victim's feelings. I have never met anyone who has not tried, usually at great personal cost, to *forget about it,* sometimes without even being fully aware of what *it* is. In the most extreme cases suicide becomes the means of *putting it in the past, just forgetting about it.* Suicide can become the final solution in escaping the *'badness'* the victim wrongly believes is at the core of their being.

Why can't you just forget about it? You are shaped by your inborn personality traits and life experiences. To suggest one should be able to forget a part of self is impossible. I'm not suggesting that you embrace your abuse and make it your identity, rather that you embrace the wounded part of self so you can heal. Understanding your abusive experiences is about knowing where you are and how you got there so *you*, not your experiences, can decide where you want to go. That is what *'getting on with it'* really means. It is through acknowledging and understanding how you have been impacted by your experiences that you are able to move beyond the distortions and faulty beliefs. Your strength, your courage, your ability to see clearly and most importantly, *to live in truth*, is dependent on facing the abuse. You need to grieve for what you lost; innocence, safety, self worth, confidence, trust, power, and the chance to grow up free of fear as any child deserves to.

"It interferes in all aspects of my life. I can't trust, I can't believe, I can't hope, I can't dream and I can't love." - C

You can't change what happened but you can change how it continues to impact you. You have a choice, you can go on surrendering your power to your abusers by continuing to live out the *lies* they told you or you can live your past in triumph by choosing to heal. The most vulnerable parts of yourself can become your greatest strengths if you allow them to be transformed through healing.

As you recover and release your self-hatred you will find you are more compassionate and empathetic toward yourself and others.

"For years I was so wrapped up in hating and judging myself as unworthy there was no room for anything else. To me people were in one of two categories, either strong or weak. Now I know we all have strengths and weaknesses. We all need caring and understanding."

Healing transforms your fears into confidence. Knowing you have faced and conquered the awful fears linked to your abuse will give you confidence in yourself and your ability to handle whatever the future might bring.

"My whole life before revolved around trying to feel safe. I was afraid of everything…afraid that if I wasn't on guard every minute of the day something bad would happen…afraid people wouldn't like me ……afraid of the pain …. afraid….afraid…. afraid. I know now, I can't always stop bad things from happening but I can take care of myself if they do."

The shame you have felt at the core of your being will disappear and pride will take its place.

"Since I came to really understand, not just in my head but in my whole being, I was not in any way responsible for the abuse the crippling guilt I felt for so long is gone. Now I'm able to look at what I've done right not just at what I believe I've done wrong. I'm proud of myself for what I've accomplished."

Only you can give yourself permission to be who you really are. Only you can decide to live out in the open, not hiding behind your defenses. No matter what others choose to do you can move forward with the confidence that comes from knowing you will always be loved, first by your Creator and secondly by yourself.

What's love got to do with it? Quite simply everything. We all need to be loved. It is the fear of losing love that keeps victim's clinging to the secret of their abuse. *"If you really knew how bad I am you wouldn't love me."*

It is the same fear that causes victim's to excuse their offenders. *"My dad drank a lot so he really didn't know what he was doing."* You can't allow yourself to think, in some instances, the very people you loved and depended on were the same ones who hurt you or allowed others to hurt you. Victims will sacrifice themselves so mom doesn't have to know her favorite brother was a molester. *"I don't want her to blame me or worse yet, hate me."* You believe the lies you're told, you believe it's some flaw within you that caused others to abuse you.

When children are abused outside the home they still fear what will happen to their families if they tell. They fear they will be blamed or not believed. This is particularly true for children who are already experiencing some form of abuse inside their home. Fear and shame keeps them silent, especially in cases of sexual abuse. *"If anyone knew how tainted I am they would be disgusted."*

Victims cannot risk losing whatever love and acceptance they believe they have. However little it might be they will hang onto it at all costs. It is what keeps them emotionally and psychologically safe and connected in the world.

Unfortunately many victims end up developing a distorted perception of what love is and as a result find themselves in abusive adult relationships.

Victims operating from a *survival mentality,* attach themselves to people or things for security. This is not love, again it is *fear.* This kind of attachment opens the door to suffering. On an unconscious level a victim may chose a partner who will either be abusive or allow themselves to be abused thus duplicating the abusive patterns of childhood. Emotional well-being becomes wholly dependent on holding onto who ever or what ever the victim has become attached to. Survivors drastically underestimate their abilities and desirability. People in survival mode will typically act out their dependency by becoming *pleasers* or *controllers.* Pleasers are afraid to say no and as a result set too few boundaries. *"I'll do what you want so you will stay attached to me."* The cost of being a pleaser is the loss of self. Controllers, on the other hand, don't hear anyone else's 'no.' They expect others to comply with their desires. *"If I stay in control of you then you will stay attached to me and give me what I want and need."* The cost of being a controller is the loss of the true joy of love that is given freely.

Authentic love honors the sacred bonds of mutuality. Authentic love is built on mutuality, mutual support, respect, empathy and concern for the well being of the other. If genuine love exists it will survive, if lost it was only an illusion to begin with. You can let go of these illusions and make room for people who will genuinely love you. Distorting a child's vision of what love is and manipulating their fear of being deprived of loving relationships is an act that ranges from depravity to irresponsibility. For example a father who has sex with his child and says he is doing it out of love is depraved. A parent who uses fear and intimidation by threatening to leave and not return, is at the very least irresponsible.

DEGREE OF TRAUMA

The severity of impact will not be the same for everyone who has been abused. The degree of trauma depends on a number of factors:

1. The relationship between the offender and the victim
2. Life circumstances before the abuse
3. Developmental stage of the victim
4. Nature of the abuse
5. Availability of supportive people

The relationship between the offender and the victim

Generally speaking the closer the relationship between the offender and the victim the greater the emotional distress will be. Children who are abused by someone they love and trust usually experience greater emotional and psychological harm. Incest by a parent is the ultimate betrayal. Even in situations where the abuser is not a member of the immediate family, but has close personal ties, the child will often feel their parents have betrayed them through their very association with the perpetrator. In some instances, particularly with younger children, the child may believe that the abuser's actions were allowed by the parent. For example how often do we instruct our children to *"Listen to the babysitter."* We even on occasion encourage our children to believe that as parents we know everything. *"If you misbehave I'll know."* The closer the biological ties between the victim and the perpetrator the more likely the abuse has occurred in the child's own home. A child's home should be a refuge, their shelter against the storm, not a place of pain and untold secrets. When a child discloses abuse and is not believed additional and equally damaging trauma is experienced.

"When I told my mother my stepfather was coming into my room at night she slapped my face and called me a liar. Even after all these years I think that's still what hurts me the most. He was a sick freak but she was my mom."

Children are completely dependent on their parents and caregivers. They rely on them, not only for the necessities of their physical life but for their emotional life as well. Parents are the yardsticks by which children measure themselves and their place in the world. If their parents reject them they believe the world will surely reject them. If their parent's are not safe or do not provide safety they believe the world must be unsafe. If their parents are unreliable they believe the world must be unreliable.

The overwhelming conclusion survivors typically reach is:

"If those who are the closest to me cannot be trusted how can I possibly trust anyone else?"

Personalize:

The relationship between me and my abuser(s) was:

_____

_____

_____

_____

_____

_____

Were my caregivers responsible in providing me with adequate protection?

_____

_____

_____

_____

_____

_____

_____

How did my abuser(s) violate my Basic Rights? (Refer to Page 18)

_____

_____

_____

_____

_____

Life circumstances before the abuse

The victim's life circumstance prior to the abuse is a key factor as it pertains to emotional resiliency and recovery. Just as a person who is physically and mentally fit has a better chance of making a full recovery from an accident so it is with the recovery of abuse. For example, in the case of sexual abuse that occurs outside the family a child who is living in an abuse free, supportive environment is in a strong position to overcome the damaging effects of abuse. A child who is living in an abusive or neglectful environment is already in a position of great vulnerability. The abuse then serves to further expand and reinforce a negative self-concept which is already taking root in the child.

There are numerous variables which will impact the manner in which trauma gets acted out in the victim's life. Previous life events, such as illness, divorce or death, physical appearance, social and financial status and natural personality traits will all influence the degree of trauma. Birth order often has a notable effect on how trauma is demonstrated through the natural personality. An excellent book on understanding the influences of birth order on shaping the personality is The New Birth Order Book by Dr. Kevin Leman. The following information has been adapted from The New Birth Order Book.

Eldest children tend to be responsible, conscientious individuals. They are natural leaders who possess good organizational skills. They are *list makers*. Eldest children often have perfectionist tendencies. And while they have high standards for others they demand even more from themselves. In fact eldest children will take on more than their share of the work rather than risk it *not being done right*. Eldest children tend to see the things they do as an extension of themselves, *"I'm only as good as what I can achieve."*

Middle children are often the mediators of the family. They typically try to avoid conflict through compromise and diplomacy. Middle children may feel they have no clear role in the family. They don't have the privileges of the eldest or the indulgences of the youngest. Middles often feel they aren't treated fairly. As a result they are typically quite independent, often finding the recognition and acceptance they need from peers. Middle children tend to be more reserved in expressing their feelings.

Youngest children like attention and are not above using charm and manipulation to get it. They are often affectionate, people orientated individuals who place more importance in talking about ideas than actually doing them. Because there wasn't much left to accomplish or be first at by the time they came along, youngest tend to develop their wit and people skills as a means of gaining recognition. They are often tenacious when it comes to getting what they want.

Only children share many of the characteristics of eldest children but super-sized. They tend to put extreme pressure on themselves to be flawless and are often black and white thinkers. They are reluctant to try new things for fear of failure. Only children may be self-absorbed, having become accustomed to being the center of their parent's world. They are often attracted to scholarly pursuits.

There are a number of factors that can influence or alter common characteristics of birth order:

- A significant age gap between siblings, five years or more, may create a second family in which the birth order repeats itself.

- Different sex siblings, the oldest of each gender possessing characteristics of an eldest child.

- Blending families through marriage or adoption.

When we explore the effects of abuse trauma it isn't difficult to envision how birth order characteristics may influence the manner in which trauma is acted out in the victim's life. Natural characteristics are often presented in extreme fashions in an attempt to regain some sense of control. Eldest children's tendencies toward perfectionism may become uncontrollable urges or phobias. Middle children, who often have difficulty expressing feelings, may lock themselves in a world of rigid emotional control, silently holding onto their grief and fear. Youngest children, who suffer abuse, may become master manipulators believing it is the only way to get the affection and recognition they need. Only children may decide they are so flawed they are no longer fit too live.

These are just a few examples of how abuse trauma can destructively interact with natural personality traits. It further illustrates how easily a victim can confuse the impact of their abusive experiences with who they are as people.

Personalize:

What is your birth order in your family?

_____

_____

_____

_____

_____

What characteristics do you possess which are common for your birth order?

_____

_____

_____

How has the abuse trauma revealed itself through your characteristics?

_____

_____

_____

Were you adopted? If yes; how may this have effected the abuse trauma?

_____

_____

_____

Were there financial hardships in your family? If yes how may this have effected the abuse trauma?

_____

_____

_____

_____

Were there physical factors that influenced you, such as illness or appearance? If yes how may have these effected the abuse trauma?

_____

_____

_____

_____

Did you experience any kind of family crisis such as death, divorce, remarriage or discord within the family? If yes how may this have effected the abuse trauma?

_____

_____

_____

_____

Degree of Trauma

Developmental stage of the victim

All human beings go through stages of psychological development. Each stage or developmental task must be successfully completed if we are to succeed at the next task. To successfully complete the developmental tasks the following conditions must be met:

- Basic needs (food, clothing, shelter) must be adequately met
- Emotional needs for love and safety must be met. These needs are met through nurturing, appropriate touch, communication and a safe environment.
- Intellectual and social needs must be met. These needs are met through stimulation (opportunities to play and to learn).

If these conditions have not been adequately and appropriately met, some form of abuse has occurred. For example if a child's basic needs (food, clothing or shelter) are not sufficiently met physical abuse in the form of neglect has occurred. If the child is inappropriately touched in a sexual way sexual abuse has occurred. If the child's emotional needs have been ignored emotional abuse has occurred.

To heighten your awareness of how you have been impacted by abuse you must understand how it interfered with the normal progression of the developmental stages. It is also important to explore any emotional vulnerability which may have existed *prior* to the abuse as these will increase the impact of the abuse trauma. For example an insecure attachment in infancy will magnify any trauma that occurs in a later developmental stage.

Questions pertaining to each developmental stage have been included to help you determine whether your needs were adequately met. You may need to do some detective work to answer the questions which relate to the first two stages. Hopefully there will be people who can provide you with information regarding these questions. If not, based on what you know about your family, make your best guess.

There are four major developmental tasks.

1. To form bonds or emotional attachments to others (Prenatal - Two Years)

Although we continue to form bonds and emotional attachments to others throughout our lives it is in infancy that we learn how to bond. In fact bonding begins in the womb. If a child is unwanted or abuse occurs in the first year of life their ability to form healthy attachments to others is impaired. Our sense of being connected to another is our emotional security in the world. It is the umbilical cord, if you will, that connects us to the human race. Without an initial strong sense of attachment we feel, to a corresponding degree, emotionally isolated, alone and unsafe in the world. Most of us are familiar with the reaction of very young infants when they are left exposed. When you remove a baby from the bath and lay him down without covering him he will panic, screaming and flailing his arms and legs. He will instinctively try to grasp something that will provide security, something to *hang onto*. The infant will remain in this agitated state until he is covered or held. So it is with those who have not successfully bonded. They are psychologically flailing, trying to hang onto something which will give them some sense of security and safety.

It is critical for a child to know their feelings are met with empathy, acceptance and are reciprocated. When this occurs the child and parent are in sync with each other. As this process of being in sync is demonstrated repeatedly the child begins to develop the sense that others share his feelings. This translates into the understanding that *"my feelings are okay"* and, *"how I feel matters."* Unfortunately parents are not always in sync with their children. The child may be **over** or **under** responded to. If for instance a particular range of emotion, such as sadness, is consistently met with a lack of empathy the child will begin to avoid expressing or even feeling that emotion. If the child's feeling is over responded to the opposite is true. The child may demonstrate a degree of feeling which is disproportionate to the situation, emotionally over responding. Children *catch* moods. For instance a three month old baby of a depressed mother will *mirror* the mother's mood, displaying more feelings of sadness and demonstrating less spontaneity and curiosity. The degree to which the infant is nurtured, emotionally and physically, corresponds with the degree of bonding which is achieved between parent and child.

Personalize:

In this first stage of development was there any form of abuse occurring in your life?

Did any major life events occur during this stage?

_____

_____

_____

_____

Were you born into a two-parent family?

_____

_____

_____

_____

Was your birth planned?

_____

_____

_____

_____

Did your mother suffer from post-partum depression?

Were you a healthy baby?

How old were your siblings at the time of your birth?

Were there other siblings born within two years after your birth?

_____

_____

_____

_____

Were your parent's affectionate to each other?

_____

_____

_____

_____

Were your parent's openly affectionate with their children?

_____

_____

_____

_____

Did you parent's over or under respond to you?

_____

_____

_____

_____

Were there other family members who spent time with you?

_____

_____

_____

_____

What kind of stories are told about you as an infant?

_____

_____

_____

_____

Was there financial stress in your family?

_____

_____

_____

_____

What feelings do you think you may have "absorbed" from your environment?

_____

_____

_____

_____

Consider your answers carefully and then summarize this developmental stage by answering the following questions:

What kind of an attachment or emotional bond do you now suspect you had with your parents - secure, moderately secure, insecure or emotionally isolated?

_____

_____

_____

Which core belief, "I am good or I am bad," do you believe was reinforced in this developmental stage?

_____

_____

_____

_____

2. To develop a sense of self (Toddler - Five Years)

The task of developing a sense of ourselves as separate beings, from those we are attached to, begins in late infancy and continues throughout the toddler years. To achieve a healthy sense of self the first developmental task of bonding must be adequately completed. We cannot form a sense of *separateness* if we have not first developed a sense of *oneness* with another. In other words we cannot separate from something if we haven't been attached to it in the first place. Do not confuse the concept of separation with the *emotional isolation* which is experienced when we are not adequately bonded. In isolation we are alone, in separateness we begin to be ourselves while remaining attached to others. *"We are ourselves but not alone."* All parents are familiar with the terrible twos. It is the period in which the child begins to strongly recognize they have their own will. "No" becomes their favorite word as they struggle to assert themselves as individuals. Part of the task of developing the *sense of self* is the identification of sex-roles. The child identifies with their parent of the same sex, learning the meaning of being a boy or a girl.

An important aspect in the healthy development of self is the way in which others, particularly parents, view and respond to the child. Children must be seen and responded to as individuals. As a means of further building a sense of identity parents need to help their children identify their specific talents and characteristics.

Personalize:

In this second stage of development was there any form of abuse occurring in your life?

_____

_____

_____

_____

Did any major life events occur during this stage?

_____

_____

_____

_____

Were you a happy child?

_____

_____

_____

_____

When did you learn to talk? / When did you learn to walk?

_____

_____

_____

Did your parent's play with you, if so how often?

_____

_____

_____

Did you have other children to play with?

_____

_____

_____

Was there a special place to play in your home?

_____

_____

_____

_____

What kind of toys did you have to play with?

_____

_____

_____

_____

Were you given praise and encouragement?

_____

_____

_____

_____

Did your parents describe you in specific ways, (funny, smart, kind)?

_____

_____

_____

_____

Did you have fears, if so how did your parent's handle them?

_____

_____

_____

How were you disciplined?

_____

_____

_____

_____

What did you learn from how you were disciplined?

_____

_____

_____

_____

Did you want to be like your parent of the same sex? If yes why, if no why not?

_____

_____

_____

_____

Consider your answers carefully and then summarize this developmental stage by answering the following questions:

What kind of a sense of self or identity do you think you developed in this stage?

"I thought I was a good kid - I really didn't know whether I was a good kid or not - I thought I was a bad kid."

_____

_____

Which core belief, "I am good or I am bad," do you believe was reinforced in this developmental stage?

3. TO DEVELOP PEER RELATIONSHIPS AND SET GOALS (SIX TO TWELVE YEARS)

This is the stage of development which occurs in the primary school years. It is during this period that children learn how to make and maintain friendships as well as learning how to set and work towards goals. Children who have not successfully completed the first and/or second developmental tasks will of course be unable to adequately accomplish this task. To be in authentic relationship with others one must have a self. **You must be in the relationship, not who you think you should be or who others want you to be.** Emotional intimacy begins with the relationship you have with yourself. If there is little or no concept of the true self any relationship formed will lack intimacy. Emotional intimacy happens only when we allow ourselves to know and be known by another. Some abused children can set goals and work independently to achieve them. However they often do not possess healthy attitudes regarding their goals. For example they may not strive to achieve for their own sense of personal satisfaction but rather because they feel they must prove to others that they have worth.

Personalize:

In this third stage of development was there any form of abuse occurring in your life?

_____

_____

_____

_____

Did any major life events occur during this stage?

_____

_____

_____

_____

Did you have friends at school?

_____

_____

_____

_____

What common interests did you share with your friends?

_____

_____

_____

Could you stand up for yourself with other children?

_____

_____

_____

Were you involved in any sports or clubs?

_____

_____

_____

How did you spend your spare time?

_____

_____

_____

What were your grades like?

_____

_____

_____

Were you given help with work you found difficult?

_____

_____

_____

What did you want to be when you grew up and why?

_____

_____

_____

_____

Did you have any goals? If so, did you receive support to meet your goals?

_____

_____

_____

_____

Consider your answers carefully then summarize this developmental stage by answering the following questions:

What kind of friendships did I have during this developmental stage? Did I feel connected to people? Did I take pride in accomplishing goals?

_____

_____

_____

_____

What core belief "I am good or I am bad," do you believe was reinforced in this developmental stage?

_____

_____

_____

_____

4. SEPARATE FROM PARENTS
(ADOLESCENCE TO EARLY ADULTHOOD)

Separating from parents is the primary task of adolescence. If children have succeeded in accomplishing the preceding developmental tasks they now possess the basic skills to undertake the final step into healthy adulthood. Parents at this stage in their children's lives should no longer be controlling the child but rather influencing and guiding their children in making good decisions. Children who are abused typically lack the ability to make good decisions for themselves. They often fail to integrate their own wants and needs with a sense of personal responsibility that assists them in setting and achieving goals. Victims may be so accustomed to being controlled by others they lack personal power to manage and direct their own lives in an affirmative manner.

Personalize:

In this fourth stage of development was there any form of abuse occurring in your life?

_____

_____

_____

_____

_____

Did any major life events occur during this stage?

_____

_____

_____

_____

What kind of goals did you set for yourself?

_____

_____

_____

_____

What kind of decisions did you make for yourself?

_____

_____

_____

_____

_____

What kind of guidelines/rules did your parents give you?

_____

_____

_____

_____

_____

What kind of responsibilities did you have?

_____

_____

_____

_____

_____

If your opinions differed from those of your parents how was that handled?

_____

_____

_____

_____

_____

Did you feel comfortable expressing your opinions? If not why not?

_____

_____

_____

_____

Consider your answers carefully then summarize this developmental stage by answering the following questions:

Did I leave home under good circumstances? Did I feel confident leaving home?

Was I looking forward to starting a life of my own or did I mostly just want to get away from the life I had at home?

_____

_____

_____

_____

Which core belief "I am good or I am bad" do you believe was reinforced in this developmental stage?

_____

_____

_____

_____

_____

_____

BOUNDARIES

It is during the developmental stages that we are building and solidifying our boundaries. Building boundaries is an integral part of the developmental process. We have invisible and visible boundaries. Our visible or outside boundary is our physical self. Our invisible or inside boundaries are the internal *fences*, emotional, spiritual, relational and sexual, which define us as being uniquely ourselves. These fences have gates that are intended to let in what is desirable and to keep out what is not.

Abuse interferes with the developmental process. It stops the child from progressing in their psychological development in a healthy way. The boundaries or *gates* of an abused child do not function effectively. They are either flung wide open for all to enter, friend and enemy alike, or slammed closed with access given to none. The two most common means by which unhealthy boundaries are demonstrated are:

1. Being overly compliant as demonstrated by:

- being unable to say no

- being afraid to disagree

- being unable to clearly state your needs, wants and feelings

2. Being overly controlling as demonstrated by:

- being unable to accept no for an answer

- using intimidation or manipulation to force others to comply

- not respecting or accepting another's person's needs, wants and feeling when they differ from their own

Personalize:

How do you think your boundaries have been influenced by the abuse?

_____

_____

_____

_____

_____

_____

_____

_____

Nature of abuse

The nature of abuse is often a critical factor in determining the degree of trauma experienced by the victim. The more intrusive and long term the abuse has been the greater the risk of increased trauma. With each incident of abuse the self-destructive emotions the victim feels deepen and become more difficult to eradicate. The degree of physical violence must also be considered. Children who are subject to brutal and relentless physical pain often display a greater degree of trauma. Abuse that includes terrorizing the child with threats of additional harm to themselves or those they love further traumatizes the child. The child will also have to cope with vivid imaginings of those threats being acted out. Through the use of pain you can teach the fiercest animal to be passive. How much more easily can a child be terrorized? The emotional pain attached to any form of abuse lingers long after the abuse is over. In the case of sexual abuse anything seen as compliance dramatically increases the trauma to the victim:

Personalize:

How long did the abuse go on?

_____

_____

_____

_____

_____

_____

Was pain or the threat of pain used?

_____

_____

_____

In the case of sexual abuse:

Did you comply because you felt it was a way to feel loved and wanted?

_____

_____

_____

_____

(If your answer is yes remember children who are denied sufficient affection and attention are vulnerable targets for sexual predators. Remember your desire for love doesn't mean you wanted to be abused.)

Did you experience some form of physical pleasure?

(If your answer is yes remember this does not mean you wanted the abuse to happen. It simply means your body responded the way it was designed to.)

_____

_____

_____

_____

_____

_____

_____

_____

Availability of supportive people

Regardless of the circumstances all of us need supportive people in our lives. Children who have support are more likely to disclose abuse than those who do not. Because a child's need for security is a critical factor for their emotional survival and well being, abuse which occurs in the home is the least likely to be disclosed by the child. However it is important to note here that many children who do have supportive family environments don't disclose abuse that occurs outside the home. Even though the child's fear of loosing their parent's love and support or fear of being blamed may be completely unfounded, the child may still feel it is a real threat. As parents it is common for us to link our children's misbehaviors with the possibility of future painful outcomes. *"If you jump on the bed you're going to fall off and hurt yourself."* Because children are conditioned in this way it is natural for them to believe they are guilty of some misbehavior which caused the abuse to happen.

When a child does disclose to an outside source it is frequently an accidental disclosure or occurs when the child is at an age where they are less dependent on the family for survival, usually adolescence. Accidental disclosure occurs when the child does not consciously decide to reveal the abuse. Typically the abuse comes to light because a third party becomes suspicious of the child's behavior or some other circumstance leads to further investigation.

How a child is responded to when they make a disclosure is crucial to the recovery process. If the child is believed and immediate action is taken to insure their safety and absolve them from blame, a significant step has already been taken. These actions say to the child *"it is not your fault and you have worth."* Psychological damage is significantly increased if the child is disbelieved, blamed, expected to act like it never happened or if someone, particularly someone the child views as a protective figure, witnessed or had knowledge of the abuse but made no attempt at intervention. It is my opinion the damage done under these circumstances can in fact be the most painful part of the abuse experience particularly if it involves a parent(s).

"My mom never tried to get help when my dad was beating up on us kids. She always made excuses for him… he was stressed out or he didn't mean it or he was sorry and just couldn't say it. She referred to his abuse as "private family business" which we were not to tell anyone about. She was always warning us not to do anything to upset him. Ironically it was my dad who decided he had enough of us and walked out on his family. I haven't seen him since I was ten years old. I don't really care, he was a lousy drunk who was unfortunately a part of my life for too long. My mom is always after me about why I don't come and visit more but to tell the truth I find it hard to be around her and control my anger. She seems oblivious to the harm done to all her children. I know she isn't the one who actually did it but she didn't do anything to make it stop. I understand she was afraid of him but we were just defenseless little kids. She was the one we counted on because she was the one who said she loved us."

It is important to note adults who disclose past or present abuse also require support. It is essential that they be *believed, absolved* and *supported* in their recovery process. It can be overwhelming when someone tells you about their abuse experience. I have heard horrendous accounts of abuse over the years and without fail I am shocked each and every time. Encouraging someone not to talk or think about their experience is not a supportive response. You don't have to be a professional to listen, care and offer compassion. These are things all of us can do. Legitimate support helps victims understand the shame they carry belongs to the abuser not to them. When a survivor discloses, they are in fact trusting you with the very essence of themselves. Hold them in gentle hands.

Personalize:

Did you have a person or people in your life that:

Accepted you?

_____

_____

_____

_____

_____

You could trust?

_____

_____

_____

_____

_____

Could and would protect you?

_____

_____

_____

_____

Would still love you if they knew?

_____

_____

_____

_____

_____

Did anyone know about the abuse? If so was any attempt made to help or were you blamed or not believed?

_____

_____

_____

_____

_____

If you told no one why not? Were you afraid there would consequences from the abuser? Did you believe you would be blamed or not believed?

_____

_____

_____

_____

_____

Writing Your Story

Putting it all together

I want to take a moment here and congratulate you on all the incredibly hard work you've done to get to this point in your healing process. As you worked through the exercises I'm sure many thoughts, feelings and memories began to surface. It's time now to put it all together. It's time to write *your story*.

Personalize:

Use your personalization exercises to help you write your story. The following sentence beginnings may also assist you with this process.

I am a victim of abuse. I remember....... It made me think............. It made me feel......

It robbed me of.................It still effects my life by........

_____

_____

_____

_____

_____

_____

PART II

Reclaiming Yourself

You Were Created to Be Who You Are

Your existence is not an accident, no matter what the circumstances of your birth or the family you grew up in, you are not a product of random chance. You were meant to be in the world, not some imitation of yourself that has been shaped by the conditions of your life. There is no doubt the abuse you suffered affected you terribly but you cannot allow it to rob you of who you are.

Being who you were created to be is not only your God-given right it is your responsibility. *The right to 'be' is the most basic of all human rights.* You don't have to justify it or earn it but you do have to claim it. Claiming it means you must first understand that you were created to be who exactly who you are. I cannot stress strongly enough how important it is that you accept this as a *truth*. We are all custom made according to our Creators' plan. Every detail of your being was planned, your physical self, talents and personality. You were made the way you were for a reason. You have a purpose and a place in this world that is uniquely your own. You cannot fulfill your purpose unless you are being who you were created to be. We all have strengths and weaknesses. We all have aspects of ourselves we need to improve on or redirect in more beneficial ways. It is not a matter of changing who you are but rather learning to use your *self* in a way that builds you, others and the world we live in. You have the *character* God created in you.

"For I know the plans I have for you, says the Lord. They are plans for good and not for evil, to give you a future and a hope."

- Jeremiah: 29 11

MAKE A COMMITMENT TO CHANGE

Up to this point your life has been about survival. You've already accomplished that, *you have survived*. As you worked through Part 1 you uncovered the lies abuse instilled in you. Now you are ready to really *live* your life, out in the open, not hiding behind the walls of your defenses. I suspect there are more than a few of you who are hyperventilating right now. The idea of living without the walls you have built around yourself can be terrifying. Face that fear down, moment by moment. Everyone can be courageous one moment at a time. I promise you if you stand still and don't run back to the familiar patterns and beliefs of victimization; you will succeed at living the life you were intended for, a life with purpose and joy. You may encounter some resistance along the way. As you change others will have to change their way of interacting with you. They may not always like it but over time they will learn to accept the changes and will gain new respect for you.

"Get over the disease to please. Understand that you cannot please everyone. Being able to disappoint others is crucial to reclaiming your life."

- Oprah Winfrey

Personalize:

Write a statement that reflects your commitment to change.

"Right now I am angry at those who have treated me so carelessly, with so little understanding and acceptance for who I am as a person. But I am also angry at myself for accepting that kind of treatment. For not standing up for myself in a way that really counted. I am making a commitment right now to change my life. To be the person I was created to be. I am done with being a victim."

Make a Commitment to Change

_____

_____

_____

_____

_____

_____

_____

_____

_____

_____

_____

_____

Understanding Power Structures

If you were brought up in an abusive home you likely grew up seeing feelings expressed through the role of abuser or the role of victim. The power structure that exists in an abusive environment consists of two kinds of power, *power over* and *power under*. The abuser is in the power over position, dominating and controlling the victim and the environment. The victim is in the power under position, being dominated and controlled. In an abusive environment there is no *personal power* structure which allows and supports the individuality and healthy emotional growth of the family members. It is not unusual for children who have come from abusive homes to set up the same style of power structure in their adult lives, either taking the power over or the power under position. Although it is commonplace to occupy only a single position in some circumstances both positions may be assumed by one person depending upon the role they are in. For example a person may be in a power under position with their spouse and simultaneously take a power over position with their children. Regardless of which power position you adopt, over, under or a combination, it is a product of the distorted thinking which comes from unresolved abuse issues. Without working through the pain and faulty beliefs of the abuse experience you will invariably perpetuate it into adulthood, assuming to some degree either the role of abuser or victim.

"What we grow up with we learn - what we learn we practice - what we practice we become."

- Anita

Personalize:

The following lists have been included to help you determine the power positions you typically adopt. Check off the characteristics which are applicable to you for each of the roles you are in: spouse, parent, child, friend, employee/employer....... Remember you may consistently assume the same power position or you may find you adopt a different power position depending on the role you are in.

Power Over:

_____ angry

_____ manipulative

_____ lacks empathy/compassion

_____ secretive

_____ hostile

_____ controlling

_____ jealous

_____ suspicious

_____ not accepting of other's feelings and opinions

_____ blames others for his/her own inappropriate behavior

_____ ridiculing

_____ judgmental

_____ irritable

_____ acts differently (nice) around other people

_____ withdraws emotionally

_____ lacks warmth

_____ critical

_____ sarcastic

_____ inflexible

Power Under:

_____ confused

_____ anxious

_____ passive

_____ apologetic

_____ frequent feelings of sadness and depression

_____ fearful

_____ guilty

_____ overly-responsible

_____ resentful

_____ stressed

_____ insecure

_____ hurt

_____ feels crazy at times

_____ frustrated

_____ overly-compliant

Personal Power:

_____ self-aware

_____ confident

_____ over all sense of well being

_____ respectful of self and others

_____ open

_____ gives and receives affection

_____ works co-operatively to solve problems

_____ empathetic

_____ accepting of others feelings and opinions

_____ positive self-image

_____ adaptable to change

_____ acknowledges and expresses feeling in an assertive manner

You no longer have to live in a *power over* or a *power under* position. Remember you have adopted these positions as a result of the unresolved abuse issues in your life and that is over. You no longer need to be afraid of taking legitimate control of your own life or allowing the others in your life to do the same. Understanding the power structures in your life is essential to reclaiming yourself. Claiming your personal power means changing what does not promote the growth of self and the growth of others. Personal power can only be achieved by you. No one else can give it to you.

"By uncovering the unconscious rules of the power game and the methods by which it attains legitimacy, we are certainly in a position to bring about basic changes."

- Alice Miller

Personalize:

Identify the power positions you assume in your various roles and describe them.

In my role of _____, I am in a _____ position.

_____

_____

_____

_____

_____

_____

_____

Developing Your Personal Power

The Power of Your Name

Reclaiming yourself and establishing personal power requires you to develop a sense of entitlement in relation to your life. As a survivor of abuse, you may have difficulty accepting the idea that you are entitled to anything. You have been devalued, your basic rights ignored and your heart broken. You had no choice or control of your situation. Now it is up to you to decide whether you will value yourself, assert your rights and mend your broken heart or continue on as a 'victim.' It is up to you to decide whether you will settle for the crumbs off the table or pull up your chair and order a ten course meal.

Personalize:

Take some time everyday just to *"be."* Find a quiet place where you feel comfortable. Close your eyes and breathe deeply, place your hand on a pulse point, allow yourself to feel the rhythm of your breath and your heartbeat. Celebrate the miracle of your body and how it works. You are alive!

Write a statement that affirms your right to exist in the world as the person you were created to be.

"I am in the world because I am meant to be here. I have value. I am going to stop being afraid. I am going to figure out who I am and what my purpose is. I am here for a reason. I have something of value to share with the world."

_____

_____

_____

_____

Understanding ourselves and learning who we are is a life long process for all of us. For abuse victims this is particularly challenging. They become so identified with their negative belief *"I am bad,"* and the roles they play, their true identity is lost. You are someone's spouse, parent, child, sibling, friend, employee....... You try to live up to what you believe are the expectations of those roles. Life becomes about *should,* to be a good wife I should...... to be a good mother I should....... You become lost in the 'shoulds', trying to be who and what you think you should be, not realizing the only person you are qualified to be is the one you already are, the one you were created to be, yourself. There is power in *calling yourself by name.* It reminds us we are someone and we have an identity of our own. You may be a spouse, a parent, daughter........ , but it is *you* who are in those roles. It is *you* who must define those roles rather than allowing the roles to define you. You are not a role, a role is what you do. Calling yourselves by name reminds you that it is *you* who must choose, take action, and responsibility for the quality of your life and the manner in which you will fulfill your roles.

Working through the first portion of this guide clarified for you that being victimized by abuse severely distorted your self image. Many of you have spent years believing the abuse symptoms you experienced defined your character. The real you has been "M.I.A." (missing in action). To know who you are starts with determining what you value. Our values are the essence of our very being. Identifying and then integrating what we value into our daily lives creates balance, self-fulfillment, confidence and contentment. Attempting to live in opposition to our values is a recipe for a life that is fraught with discontent, frustration and emotional and mental agitation.

Personalize:

The following list of values has been included to help you discover who you are. Make your own list, choosing those which apply to you and adding any others that may not included on this list.

God	Knowledge	Self-control
Family	Wisdom	Balance
Friendship	Spirituality	Accomplishment
Community	Teaching	Competition
Service	Creativity	Serenity
Work	Solitude	Cleanliness
Security	Independence	Organization
Structure	Honesty	Learning
Physical Fitness	Integrity	Fairness
Fun	Acceptance	Connection
Adventure	Compassion	
Nature	Kindness	
Passion	Trustworthiness	

My values are:

_____

_____

_____

_____

_____

_____

_____

_____

_____

_____

_____

_____

_____

The next step is integrating your values into your daily life. This is essential if you are to live a satisfying, well balanced life. Honoring *all of our values* is synonymous with honoring ourselves. It is not enough to honor only the values we believe are acceptable to the other people in our lives. Too often we interpret differences in values as being right or wrong. There are value differences in all relationships, for instance one partner may have a strong value of community and the other partner an equally strong value of solitude, each person can easily interpret their partner's value as *being wrong.* In truth neither person is right or wrong, they are simply different. In healthy relationships participants avoid making judgments about the other's way of being. Honoring the values of both individuals, *individuals* being the operative word here, means striking a balance which leaves room for both people to be who they are. Being in a relationship with someone who is unwilling to honor your values certainly makes it more difficult to live a value based life. But it does not make it impossible. Don't wait for someone to give you permission to be who you are. You're the only person who can do that. Living your values means living out in the open, where the world can see the real you. Most of us are familiar with the biblical quote, *"Do not hide your light under a bushel."* It appears in the bible, not only once, but in three of the Gospels, Matthew, Mark and Luke. Obviously this is a lesson that our Creator wanted to be sure we all understood. Your "light" has been created especially for you by God. All that He creates is right and good so let your light shine!

Personalize:

Fear is the number one barrier to living an authentic life. Fear that you will once again be vulnerable to being hurt in some way. Think about the fears stopping you from being your authentic self. To help you identify your barriers the following list of questions has been included for you to consider. Answer the questions which ring true for you as honestly as you can.

What if others reject the "real" me?

What will happen if I stop trying to please everybody?

What if people don't like what I have to say?

_____

_____

_____

_____

_____

What if they don't approve of the decisions I make?

_____

_____

_____

_____

_____

What will they do if I disagree with them?

_____

_____

_____

_____

Will they think I'm being selfish if I say no?

_____

_____

_____

_____

What if I stop rescuing everyone?

_____

_____

_____

_____

_____

_____

If people no longer need me to look after them will they still value me?

_____

_____

_____

_____

_____

What if I stop being so busy I actually have time to face my true feelings?

_____

_____

_____

_____

_____

Who will I be if I'm no longer a victim?

_____

_____

_____

_____

_____

Will there be things I will have to take responsibility for if I'm no longer a victim?

_____

_____

_____

_____

_____

Will I have to stop trying to make other people responsible for my well-being?

_____

_____

_____

_____

_____

What would happen if I saw myself as an equal in my relationships?

_____

_____

_____

_____

_____

What would happen if I clearly stated what I need from my relationships?

_____

_____

_____

_____

_____

_____

What would happen if I stopped manipulating others to meet my needs?

_____

_____

_____

_____

_____

What if I stopped trying to impose my will onto others?

_____

_____

_____

_____

_____

What if I stopped taking all the responsibility for the well being of my relationships?

_____

_____

_____

_____

What if I stopped blaming myself every time someone has a conflict with me?

_____

_____

_____

_____

What if I stopped blaming someone else every time someone has a conflict with me?

_____

_____

_____

_____

_____

What if I demanded that my basic rights be respected?

_____

_____

_____

_____

_____

What if I refused to tolerate being abused in any way?

_____

_____

_____

_____

What if I stopped abusing others?

_____

_____

_____

_____

Giving into fears that stop you from being authentically you is self-rejection. You can become so afraid of the possibility of being rejected by others you reject yourself first. You do this by not honoring your own wants, needs and values. When you do this what you are really saying is other's needs and wants are more important than your own. You are saying you don't have as much worth as others. You are taking the beautiful gift of the "self" God gave only to you and handing it back unopened. Making yourself a priority is not selfish. That's not to say we don't have a responsibility to others, of course we do. The key is finding a healthy balance between meeting your own needs and being in service to others. How will you know when you have struck the right balance for you? You will have a greater sense of contentment and peace of mind. You will feel free from having to make excuses or justify your decisions. You will be able to tolerate others disagreeing with you and allow them to have their own opinion without feeling you have to change your own, or theirs. Building your life on your values will give you the solid foundation you need to live your life in truth. Make it your intention to live your values everyday.

Personalize:

Take a moment and write out a statement of intention. It is a good idea to write out your intentions frequently. It will help you to stay focused and moving toward your goals.

"It is my intention to stop trying to live life based on other people's expectations of whom or what I should be. Instead I will live my life based on my own values and my own expectations and goals. I am no longer willing just to be absorbed into the lives of those around me. I will live a life that is my own. ...."

Take some time to reflect on your list of values. Hopefully you now have a greater sense of clarity in relation to; who you are, what changes you want to make in your life and what goals you want to set for yourself. Now that you have a better understanding of what your values are and the barriers preventing you from living a self-directed life let's look at how this is currently reflected in your daily living. Start with the values that are the most important to you. Once you have integrated them into your daily life add a few more and so on until you are living a value based life.

Personalize:

List the various roles you have in your life. (spouse, parent, child, sibling, friend, employee......)

Beneath each one write how each of your values is presently reflected in the role.

Next write down any barriers that may be getting in the way of fully integrating your values into your roles.

Write down an action you will take which will bring your values into those roles.

Finally write down how you believe this action will improve your life.

Role:

My value of _____, *is currently reflected in this role by:*

_____

_____

_____

_____

_____

My barriers to fully integrating this value are:

_____

_____

_____

_____

_____

I am going to more fully integrate this value by taking action. I will:

_____

_____

_____

_____

_____

Taking this action will improve my life by:

_____

_____

_____

_____

_____

Continue the above process for each of your roles:

_____

_____

_____

_____

_____

Are your values reflected in your environment?

Your environment also plays a part in how your values are reflected in your life. To help you identify the type of environment which would contribute to your sense of well being answer the following questions.

Personalize:

List three words that describe your most desirable feeling states?

_____

_____

_____

Are these feeling states reflected in your environment? If yes, how?

_____

_____

_____

_____

_____

_____

What is your favorite season and why?

_____

_____

_____

_____

Are any of the attributes of your favorite season reflected in your environment?

If yes, how? If no, how can you include them?

_____

_____

_____

_____

_____

REPROGRAMMING YOUR THINKING THROUGH THE POWER OF LANGUAGE

Language is powerful. In part what we think is programmed by what we hear. As a victim of abuse you most likely have been the recipient of critical, harsh words. In turn your own internal voice becomes an echo of the same kind of verbalizations.

"My father was always saying things like, "why are you so stupid?,....... can't you do anything right?.......I say the same things to myself every time I think I've made a mistake."

Changing the negative language we use to positive language breaks the old destructive programming. Use strong words to stop your punitive internal voice whenever you hear it. *"Stop! It's not true! I will not verbally abuse myself!"*

Whatever words work for you are fine. Immediately follow up any negative talk with an affirming statement countering the negativity that robs you of confidence and self-esteem. *"I am intelligent! I am allowed to make mistakes! I'm worth it! I am a good person!"*

Even if your affirming statements sound false at first keep repeating them. Remember you are not only deprogramming yourself you are simultaneously reprogramming your thinking and feeling. You are learning to treat yourself with respect. You are changing how you perceive yourself and consequently how others perceive you. Your words effect the way you feel about yourself and that in turn effects how others perceive you. If your declarations are tentative even apologetic you will be perceived as an indecisive, uncertain person. When you speak with conviction and confidence you will be perceived as a person of conviction and confidence.

POWER-ROBBING WORDS, PHRASES AND HABITS

- **Using words like should and ought.** These words rob you of your power and instill guilt. Make a point of using phrases instead that reinforces your power to choose what you do. Eliminate these words from your vocabulary.

Disempowering Statement: *"I really should volunteer for the school committee but I don't know where I could find the extra time."*

Empowering Statement: *"I choose not to volunteer for the school committee. I don't have the extra time."*

- **Over - apologizing.** When you constantly apologize for things you can't control you automatically put yourself in a one-down position. It conveys the message that you have done something wrong.

Disempowering Statement: *"I'm sorry I'm very emotional about this. I'm sorry if it makes you uncomfortable."*

Empowering Statement: *"I know discussing this makes you uncomfortable but I have very strong feelings that I need to express."*

- **Over - explaining.** When you over-explain and justify you are in fact conveying you need permission and approval, that you lack confidence in your own perceptions or decisions.

Disempowering Statement: *"I'm thinking about taking a day for myself. I will have time to clean the house tonight and the kids are going to be out for part of the tomorrow anyway."*

Empowering Statement: *"I am taking a day for myself tomorrow."*

- **Asking for permission instead of making a statement.** Of course there are times when asking is appropriate but that certainly does not apply to every situation.

Disempowering Statement: *"The leaves need to be raked." Do you think you kids could make time to help me this week-end?"*

Empowering Statement: *"Please make time to help me rake the leaves this week-end."*

- **Not being able to accept a compliment.** This conveys that you don't believe you are worthy of the praise given and you do not place value on yourself.

Disempowering Statement: *"I can't really take too much credit for the report. I had excellent reference material."*

Empowering Statement: *"Thank you. I'm pleased with the report."*

- **Making self-depreciating remarks.** Being able to laugh at yourself is one thing; putting yourself down is quite another. Making disparaging remarks about yourself is often a way of deflecting anticipated criticism from others for what you perceive as your short comings. Basically you are putting yourself down before someone else has the chance to. When you indulge in this habit you are diminishing yourself and your worth and you are teaching others to do the same.

Disempowering Statement: *"Oh I'm such an idiot." I'd forget my head if it wasn't screwed on. You'll just have to forgive me."*

Empowering Statement: *"I'm sorry I forgot."*

Personalize:

Take a moment to write down the negative words and statements you use most often. Beneath each one write a replacing affirmative word or statement. Take this a step further and keep a small notebook with you, making note on a daily basis of the negative words and disempowering statements you use. At the first available moment write an affirming or empowering replacement statement next to them. Review these often. Writing things down creates greater awareness of how often you slip back into old destructive programming.

The negative words and statements I use most often are:

_____

_____

_____

_____

OWNING YOUR FEELINGS

"We live in a secret place. Where thoughts and feelings are sometimes even secret from ourselves. We cannot say with honesty who we really are for that must be kept secret too."

As a victim of abuse you learned your feelings were not important. In fact you probably learned feelings are dangerous and confusing. The truth is your feelings are neither right nor wrong, they are just feelings. Most of us have been conditioned, to some degree, that certain feelings should not be expressed or even felt. Those are the feelings we don't like, the ones that are uncomfortable, the ones that make us feel out of control or the ones we believe other people won't want to hear. There is no feeling that is *wrong*. Feelings are natural reactions to situations that occur in our lives. They serve the valuable purpose of warning us when we need to change something. Acknowledging our feelings doesn't mean we have to act on them or even share them. When you experience any intense feeling it is a good idea to take some time to process it before you act. Sometimes sharing your feelings is unnecessary, you may think it through and resolve the issue on your own. There will be other times when your feelings must be expressed. Sometimes we need to vent our feeling to someone we trust, who will listen and not judge. Taking a *time out* allows you to regain emotional control and decide the best way to handle your feelings. You are responsible for your feelings and how you express them.

Of all of the emotions to deal with, many survivors state anger is the most difficult to own. For that reason I am including the following information which specifically addresses anger.

RELEASING YOUR ANGER

Go back and read through your story. Allow yourself to feel the anger that comes from fully acknowledging and understanding what being abused has cost you. It can be very difficult to get past the idea that anger is a bad thing and should not be expressed. The truth is the expression of anger is an essential part of the healing process. Expressing your anger in an honest, constructive way, releases it. It restores your power and allows you to see the truth, setting you free from guilt, self-blame and feelings of unworthiness. Holding your anger in results in bitterness, resentment, depression, physical problems and robs you of peace. You cannot wish your anger away. It is there and if you don't direct to where it belongs it you will either internalize it or displace it, directing it to places it doesn't belong. But either way you will remain emotionally attached to and directed by the abuse. You can start directing your anger appropriately by writing an 'angry letter' to each of your abusers as well as to those who didn't protect or help you. Don't worry about editing what you say, these letters will not be sent. The sole purpose of an angry letter is to give you the chance to express yourself openly and honestly without fear of losing control and damaging yourself or others.

A cautionary note here, if you find yourself entertaining thoughts of self-harm or of harming others be sure to access your support people to help you through this process.

Personalize:

Dear:

I am really angry with you. You abused me. You did .... *You made me feel*........

_____

_____

_____

_____

_____

_____

_____

_____

_____

_____

_____

EFFECTIVELY EXPRESSING YOUR FEELINGS

As your sense of your own value increases your personal power will increase likewise. How you communicate your feelings is directly related to the degree of personal power you experience in your life. When you acknowledge and respect your feelings you teach others to do the same. Expressing your feelings is not always easy. Most of us have experienced fear of being hurt, rejected and/or misunderstood. Frustrations and uncertainties are, to a certain extent, a part of all relationships. At times we have all let ourselves and others down. None of us are infallible, we are all fragile and we are all vulnerable. These things are part of the human condition. But each time you take the risk of speaking the *truth in love* you are setting yourself free and opening the door for the other person to do the same. Speaking the truth in love simply means you have the best intentions for yourself and the best intentions for the other. Even when the other person does not respond in the way you hope for, speaking in a manner that honors yourself and others will heighten your sense of self-confidence, self-respect and integrity. Each time you succeed in speaking the truth your fear and anxiety will be reduced.

COMMUNICATING WITH PERSONAL POWER

- **Express your feeling clearly without being excessively emotional.**

Expressing your feelings when you are highly emotional often results in others responding to your emotional state rather than the content of your words. This makes you exceedingly vulnerable to falling into old disempowering patterns.

- **Be willing to openly share your feelings, your hopes and dreams and encourage others to do the same.**

Relationships are built on the exchange of information. Emotional intimacy develops in relationships when we hear and empathize with the other's feelings. Empathy involves trying to understand what it feels like to be the other person, trying to see the world through their eyes. Even in those instances when we have to ask questions to clarify what the other person is saying we are building intimacy. Asking questions like, "I'm not sure what you mean could you explain it to me again?" demonstrates to the other that our intention is to understand. The degree of intimate information exchanged should correspond with the nature of the relationship. The type of personal information exchanged in a healthy spousal relationship for example, will differ from the type of information shared with a co-worker.

- **Respect other's different interests and points of view and expect others to respect yours.**

Someone disagreeing or expressing an opposing point of view does not make them your adversary. It simply means they are different from you with their own way of experiencing situations and their own feelings. No one is entitled to deny the reality and experience of the other. No one is entitled to trivialize or undermine what is of value to another.

- **Do not give or accept: accusations, blame or judgments.**

Simply state your feelings without accusing, blaming or judging the other. When we fall into these behaviors we are assuming we know what the other person's intention was. Just because for example you felt embarrassed by something someone said to you does not necessarily mean it was their *intention* to embarrass you. Accusing, blaming and judging create a vicious, frustrating cycle. The recipient becomes defensive and accuses, blames and judges in return. State your feelings and specifically ask for what you want and allow the other to do the same. This opens the door to negotiation and ultimately resolution.

EVALUATING YOUR RELATIONSHIPS

The quality of the relationships you have with others will be a reflection of the relationship you have with yourself. The quality of the relationship you have with yourself will be a reflection of the relationship you have with your Creator.

We were created for relationships. All of life is made up of relationships. We have relationships with everything: people, pets, food, substances, places, possessions and even beliefs.

Up until now your relational style has been as a victim of abuse, strongly influenced by the adults who were around you as a child. And as a victim you have been highly susceptible to a psychological pattern called *repetition compulsion*. This refers to the compulsive repetition of the feeling states, thinking patterns and behaviors that developed as a result of the abuse. In this manner the original trauma is carried forward and is reproduced in your current relationships. This happens, not because you wish to relive the pain but rather because you wish to change it and bring it to a different, more satisfying conclusion. There are those that claim every key relationship we have is, in fact, a reflection of the relationship we had with one or both of our parents and until we resolve the conflicts inherent to those primary relationships we will continue to reproduce it in the present.

By identifying these self-defeating patterns you can move forward and make positive changes instead of being forever doomed to repeat the past. It is important to remember you can never *change* the original trauma. You can't go back and rewrite your history but you are beginning to understand how you have been influenced. You are learning how to let go of the abusive patterns of the past.

"My father was emotionally unavailable. He was powerful and controlling. He could withdraw his love at a moments notice whenever you deviated from his agenda. There was one opinion, one way of doing things, one way of being and that was his way. I lived in constant fear of being thrown out of the family figuratively speaking. I learned to be quiet. It was safer to be in the background where there was less chance of being noticed and found lacking in some way which would earn his disapproval. Oddly enough I grew up and married the same kind of man. I'm still trying to figure out how to be good enough to get approval and acceptance."

"My life is completely falling apart. My wife has left me and taken our three children. She says she is sick of doing it alone, that I am never there for her or the kids. I thought I was doing the right thing by working as much as I do. I know I have been a good provider. In my family I was always

the one who was "lazy," the one who was never going to amount to anything. I guess I have spent my whole life trying to prove my old man wrong. I ended up losing my family because of it."

"I never say no to my kids. They pretty much get and do whatever they want. When we were kids our mother always threatened to leave my sister and me if we upset her. I'm afraid if my kids get upset with me they will stop loving me."

"When my mom married my stepfather he made it clear right from the beginning that I wasn't his kid. He never spoke to me unless it was to give me hell. It was pretty clear he thought I was a loser because he was really nice to his own kids, even other people's kids. I had a lot of trouble with authority figures. To this day I freak out if I think someone is criticizing me or trying to control me which gets me in trouble all over again"

It's important to remember that although the manner in which someone may choose to live their life may effect you, their choices are a reflection of them not of you or your worth. Don't make decisions based on what you think you know about the other person but rather make your decisions based on what you know about yourself. In this way you eliminate speculating on or making judgments on another person's thoughts, feeling or motivations.

"My husband is always accusing me of having an affair. Whenever I try to talk to him about something that's bothering me he responds by saying I'm just looking for an excuse to leave the marriage. I used to be so hurt when he would say those things. I couldn't believe he thought I was a liar and someone who couldn't be trusted. I finally stopped trying to convince him I'm not the kind of person. I realized the only time the accusations came up was when I needed something emotionally from him. I don't know why he does this, but for whatever reason he refuses to take any responsibility for the emotional part of our marriage. Now I understand his behavior is a result of his own issues. I have decided to leave the marriage. I will no longer participate in any relationship in which who and what I am is not recognized and respected."

Your Relationship with Your Creator

I believe the connection you have with God is the single most important factor in living a secure and satisfying life. Victims of abuse frequently describe feeling lost and alone. Life seems futile and empty. If this describes you I have good news. The good news is if you know you are lost then you already know you need to be found. That's the beginning of living in your spirit. The great news is you have never been lost to God. Not for one moment has He lost track of you, you are far too important to Him. When you are connected to your Creator you stop being lost, you are never alone and life has meaning and purpose.

This is often a difficult concept for abuse survivors. Many report feeling abandoned by God. Frequently they blame God for what has happened to them. Some victim's decide they must have offended God in some way and the abuse was their punishment. Still others conclude that God does not exist.

"If God is so good and all powerful where was He when I was being abused? I prayed and asked him to make it stop but He never answered."

In this manner the lie of abuse robs the victim of a satisfying personal relationship with their Creator. The victim is left, not only with a distorted image of self but also with a distorted image of God. All human beings have free will. Sadly, as a victim of abuse, you know only too well that there are those who choose to use their free will in terrible ways. There are six key steps in developing your relationship with your Creator.

1. Acknowledge there is a power greater than you, the Source of all creation

2. Acknowledge your Creator only wants what is good for you

3. Acknowledge your Creator can and will transform all of your life experiences into something powerful to be used for growth and goodness, if you ask.

4. Acknowledge, like all relationships, you must spend time communicating if you want a real relationship which will grow and deepen in love and trust.

5. Acknowledge you were created to be exactly who you are.

6. Acknowledge you are unconditionally loved by your Creator.

I Sat Upon a Hill

I sat upon a hill and felt God's touch in the breeze that moved my hair

I sat upon a hill and smelt God in the sun warmed grass beneath my feet

I sat upon a hill and saw God in the blueness of the sky stretched above me

I sat upon a hill and heard God's voice in a bird's song

I sat upon a hill, a hill that God had made

I breathed the air He created with the lungs that He gave me

I felt the heart He had placed in me beat with life and love

I sat upon a hill and knew I was meant to be just as I am

The degree of mutual satisfaction in a relationship can be measured by the extent to which it meets the needs of the two people involved.

Evaluate your current significant relationships. Pay particular attention to any areas where you may still be attempting to resolve original trauma. This compulsion may be easily identifiable in your life or it may be very subtle. Before you begin go back and review the work you did in Part I on *Identifying Distorted Thinking*. In Part I you looked at how your beliefs and subsequent thoughts and feelings influence your environments, home, work and social. Now you are going to look at how they specifically impact your relationships. The following questions have been included to help you. Repeat this set of questions for each of your significant relationships.

Personalize:

In my relationship with _____:

Do I feel accepted and valued for who I am?

If not, why not?

_____

_____

_____

_____

Have I experienced this before?

_____

_____

_____

_____

How will I know I am accepted and valued?

_____

_____

_____

_____

_____

_____

Do I feel appreciated for what I do?

If not, why not?

_____

_____

_____

_____

_____

Have I experienced this before?

_____

_____

_____

_____

_____

How will I know I am appreciated?

_____

_____

_____

_____

_____

Do I feel satisfied with the amount of physical/verbal affection?

If not, why not?

_____

_____

_____

_____

_____

Have I experienced this before?

_____

_____

_____

_____

How will I know when I have enough physical/verbal affection?

_____

_____

_____

_____

_____

Do I feel comfortable to openly talk about my thoughts and feelings?

If not, why not?

_____

_____

_____

_____

Have I experienced this before?

_____

_____

_____

_____

How will I know when I am comfortable to talk about my thoughts and feelings?

_____

_____

_____

_____

In the space provided below repeat the above questions for each of your significant relationships.

_____

_____

_____

EVALUATING YOUR RELATIONSHIPS

To break old destructive patterns you need to first identify them. Now that you have completed the questions for each of your significant relationships take some time and compare your answers. Do any themes or similarities emerge that mirror the feelings, thoughts and behaviors that accompanied your *original trauma?*

In all or most of my relationships I feel....... I think.........I behave...............

_____

_____

_____

_____

_____

_____

_____

_____

_____

_____

The Ten Commandments of Good Relationships

Although relationships are based on the unique combination of personality traits possessed by the two people involved, there are still some basic rules which will enhance any relationship.

1. Do unto others as you would have them do unto you

In all circumstances treat others as you would like them to treat you. Not only does this insure your personal integrity will remain intact, regardless of how others may chose to respond, but in doing so you release powerful healing energy into your relationships.

2. Speak the truth in love

Be true in what you say and remember the desired outcome is to promote well-being not only in yourself but in the other.

3. In times of disagreement don't attack the other person's character

Keep your focus on the issue. Speak from the perspective of your own thoughts and feelings. Character assassination is not only destructive, it's abusive.

4. Have a "Hallmark Moment" everyday

The power of "little acts," of kindness, appreciation and affection is seriously underestimated. These little acts tell us we are loved and valued. Choose acts that are meaningful to the other person.

5. To err is human, to forgive divine

The fruits of non-forgiveness are anger, resentment and bitterness. Forgiveness sets us free to make our choices unencumbered by these crippling emotions. Forgiveness does not mean forgetting, it doesn't mean we aren't accountable for the wrongs we do, and it doesn't mean we have to tolerate behavior that isn't acceptable.

6. Understand there are two *different* people in a relationship

Different people have different needs. We do not all think, feel and want the same things. It is critically important in any relationship to understand the other's needs are as important as your own even if they are not the same as your own. Other than behaviors that violate our basic rights there is not a right and wrong, there is only 'different.' The key is to work together to accommodate the needs of both people. Our differences can in fact enhance our relationships. Each person can gain from learning from the other's differences.

7. Think of your relationship as a living thing.

Your relationships are alive. They change and grow. Like all living things relationships need care; without it they wither and they die.

8. Be present, emotionally, physically and spiritually

Relationships require the active participation of both people involved. Love is a verb: an action word. It is not enough just to say you care for the other you must show that care by meaningful action. Emotionally anaesthetizing yourself with busy work; food, television, shopping or whatever your drug of choice is not a solution to life's stresses and challenges. Be *involved* in your relationships.

9. Nurture growth in each other

Our relationships should provide us with a safe place to grow, to challenge ourselves to be our best *self* and to encourage the other to do the same. That doesn't mean telling the other what is wrong with them but rather offering them support to explore and develop their potential. Relationships should never be a competition with somebody winning and somebody losing. It is within our relationships we can become our *best self.*

10. Have fun together

Laughter can indeed be the best medicine. Too often we get so caught up in the demands of daily living we forget to stop and just enjoy ourselves. Just because you're grown up doesn't mean you don't need to play.

Personalize:

How do you, or will you, live these relationship rules in your life?

Based on your values include some of your own relationship rules.

_____

_____

_____

_____

_____

_____

_____

_____

_____

Confronting Your Abusers

Confronting your abusers is a necessary step in bringing closure to those relationships which have caused you so much pain. The purpose of confrontation is to take back your legitimate power. Confronting your abusers breaks the pattern of victimization. It is important to note here confronting is not the same as attacking. Confronting is simply stating the *truth*, the truth being; the facts and feelings associated with your abuse. Do not confront with the expectation of getting anything from your abuser. If regaining your power depends on whether or not your abuser accepts the truth and is genuinely remorseful for the suffering they have caused, you will quite possibly remain in the position of victim. Unfortunately the reality is the victim often does not get the validation they want. Confrontation is not about "getting them to accept responsibility," confrontation is really about "getting yourself free." Free to either end the relationship or try and resolve it. Free to move forward and embrace your life, not as it was then but how you will live it now.

There are a number of ways you can confront your abuser; face-to-face, in a letter, by telephone or by e-mail. If a real-life confrontation is not an option, you can still experience emotional release through alternate means. You can write a letter and not mail it, you can imagine a scenario in which you successfully confront your abuser or you can conceive your own ritual. It is important to note here if you choose an alternate method be sure you are making this choice from a position of strength not fear. If direct confrontation would cause you emotional or physical harm chose an alternate method. Regardless of the method you chose be prepared to feel some anxiety. Confrontation may be one of the more unpleasant things you do in your life but it is also one of the most empowering.

"Every time you meet a situation, though you think at the time it is an impossibility and you go through the tortures of the damned, once you have met it and lived through it, you will find that forever after you are freer than you were before." - Eleanor Roosevelt

When you confront your abusers it is important to remember everything you have learned thus far about developing your personal power. Remember who you are, use the power of language, own your own feelings and effectively express them, claim your basic rights and remember what the abuse taught you about yourself is a lie.

Personalize:

Practice your confrontation by writing it down. Include the facts of what happened to you and how you felt. An example has been provided to help you with this process.

Mom:

I am angry at you for emotionally abusing me. You treated me like I didn't matter, that I was of no importance. It never occurred to me you could be wrong. If you treated me like I was nothing then it must be so. I believed that for most of my life. I allowed people to walk all over me from grade school on into my adult life. I allowed myself to be abused by others because I didn't believe I deserved anything more. You made me feel worthless. I could never talk to you about anything of importance because you always had this way of making me feel that if I was a stronger or a better person it wouldn't be happening to me. You never gave any kind of encouragement or praise so I believed I didn't deserve either. You diminished me so I diminished myself. Everything was about you, how you felt, what you didn't have, what you had to put up with. You never chose how I might feel over your own feelings. In other words you never chose me. If I felt angry with you I felt guilty, if I made a mistake I felt guilty. I felt guilty all the time in fact there was a time I felt guilty for even being alive. You think you know who I am but you don't. How could you? You've never taken the time to find out. You decided who I was a long time ago and no matter what I say or do, you never waiver from what you think is true. Whether you deny it or not these are my feelings and this is the truth about how your emotional neglect effected me.

_____

_____

_____

_____

_____

FORGIVENESS

"Take the first step in faith. You don't have to see the whole staircase just take the first step."

- Martin Luther King Jr.

You are now ready for the last remaining steps you have to take toward forgiveness. This is often a slow and difficult process. You accomplish it one step at a time. You could not truly forgive until you understood what you were forgiving. You have done that now. You have acknowledged the abuse in your life. You have identified its lies and how you have been effected by them. You now know you are not "bad," that the shame and guilt you carried was your abuser's not yours. You are aware of the symptoms and coping strategies you experienced that disguised themselves as your personality. You have expressed your anger at the injustice done to you and in some form or other you have confronted your abuser. You know you are strong, you know you are entitled to the life you were created to have. Forgiveness is the final step which allows you to let go of your identity as a victim. You are ready to let go of that identity.

Forgiveness may be the single most important factor in reclaiming yourself. Forgiveness of yourself and of those who have harmed you. Forgiveness does not mean forgetting, you will always remember. Forgiveness does not mean you are excusing the acts of abuse. You are forgiving those who have abused you. Although they will always bear the responsibility for their abusive actions, what you are forgiving is their inability to love, care, and nurture or protect you. No amount of suffering, no amount of anger, guilt, resentment, bitterness, hatred or self-condemnation can ever change what happened. Each time you experience those feelings you are victimized all over again, reliving all the suffering that was inflicted on you. There is no hope that what happened in the past can ever be changed. Let go of that futile hope and move forward unencumbered to what can be changed, your present and your future. Forgiveness is the key that opens the door of the emotional prison you have been in. Non-forgiveness keeps you miserable, with no hope that your future can be different than your past. You continue to relive the abusive relationships, you continue be the victim of your abuser. When you forgive you release yourself from past burdens.

"If you are going to seek revenge, you had better dig two graves."

- Chinese Proverb

Forgiveness is not something that just happens. To forgive is a conscious choice. It depends wholly on you. There are no prerequisites. Forgiveness can happen in the absence of any form of compensation or validation of your pain. You may never receive any acknowledgment of wrong doing from those who have harmed you but you can forgive them anyway. You can release yourself from the never ending cycle of pain and suffering that keeps you bound to your abusers. Nurture forgiveness within yourself, don't try to force it. It will bloom in its own time. Your task now is simply to prepare the ground and plant the seeds.

"Forgiveness is not for the forgiven but for the sake of the forgiver."

- Anonymous

Make a conscious decision to want to forgive everyday.

Develop the *habit* of forgiveness. Each repetition of "I want to forgive," strengthens the habit of forgiveness. Whether you are actually ready to forgive or not the very act of wanting to forgive is freeing. The desire to forgive unfailingly leads to growth of heart and spirit. Forgiveness releases the wisdom which exists in your spirit, the wisdom which leads you back to the person you were created to be. Non-forgiveness keeps you connected in a negative way to those who have hurt you.

Today I want to forgive (name your abuser or yourself). It is enough for now that I want to forgive.

Consciously release your painful feelings.

Don't expect this to happen easily or quickly. Don't delude yourself into thinking forgiveness is accomplished through pushing the feelings and thoughts back under. Observe the thoughts and feelings as they pass through your consciousness and then release them. Do not fall back into the trap of *identifying* yourself by the feelings you are experiencing. Remember you are not the abuse, you are you.

I release myself from the (name your feeling) that is filling me right now. I claim the space inside of myself for (name the feelings you want to have)

I release you (name your abuser) and all that you did to dishonor me. I release your distorted thinking, insecurities, your inability to nurture and your cruelty from my mind, from my heart and from my spirit. I leave the judgment of your wrong doing in the hands of your Creator.

LIVING FROM YOUR SPIRIT

There are two distinct ways of being, ego-centered and spirit-centered. The ego operates in the external world. Its primary function is survival of the self as it (self) is perceived from your experiences, faulty beliefs, distorted thinking and fears. As a victim of abuse it is likely you have identified yourself mainly with a self-image of someone who is less than what and who you really are. The ego becomes completely self-absorbed in its struggle to meet its perceived need for self-protection and self-sufficiency. Remember this *perceived* need has been based on faulty self-perception. You had no concept of yourself other than the *image* of self that rose from your fear and pain. When self-image is distorted it follows the images of those you have relationships with will also be distorted. You live your life in *survival mode* functioning from ego and detached from your spirit.

The following example depicts the distorted image the abuse victim has of his wife. The victim incidentally was raised by a controlling, critical parent.

"I often have strong feelings of jealousy and mistrust. I find it hard to believe my wife loves me even though we have been together for over fifteen years. When she tells me she loves me I wonder what she really wants. I feel angry with her a lot of the time but I don't talk to her about it. I think if she really loved me she would know how I feel. She keeps telling me things have to change. She says she needs me to talk to her more and get more involved in our life and on and on. I just think she is criticizing me and so we fight. She just wants to control me. No one is going to tell me I have to change. I'm good enough the way I am. No one is going to control me."

Your spiritual self is the essence of who you were created to be. It is the sacred facet of your being, presenting itself in the world as part of the grace and beauty of creation. It is the place within you where you live in unison with your Creator. The place in which you connect with the awesome peace which comes from being connected to your Source. Nothing that is not of God; in other words only what is pure and good can exist in the spirit. The spirit does not concern itself with image. Truly living in the spirit means stripping away the masks you wear for protection and security. It removes the pressure of creating and presenting what you believe is an acceptable image. A spirit-centered life focuses on building an internal world based on, what Father Paul Keenan in his book, *Stages of the Soul* refers to as hallmarks of the soul: honesty, love, beauty, goodness, freedom and service. These are the universal core values that when practiced will unfailingly connect you to your Creator, the source of all power and wisdom, and subsequently to your purpose.

Regardless of what the *specifics* of your particular purpose are and how it presents itself in the external world, we all share a common purpose. It is simply to put forth into the world only that which is good. This does not require you to have any special talents or skills, nor does it require you to be anything or anyone other than what and who you are. The wisdom of the spirit, which exists within each person, will direct the goodness you put forth in the way it is meant to go. There is no magic secret to accessing your wisdom. In fact it is very simple. ***Form the intention to put forth into the world that which is good*** and the wisdom and resources you need to accomplish your purpose will present themselves. When we place ourselves in union with our Creator we also become the recipients of His limitless resources. This does not necessarily mean material resources. Perhaps the resource we need in a particular circumstance is compassion or determination.

When you find yourself in a situation in which you are unsure ask yourself, *"What is my intention right now?"* Your intention will be either ego-based or spirit based. Is it some form of self-interest which is motivating you? If it is there will be accompanying feelings which do not exist in the spirit; fear, resentment, bitterness, anger, greed......just to name a few. Is it motivated by love and a desire to bring forth that which is good? Are the *hallmarks* of the soul present, honesty, love, beauty, goodness, freedom and service?

"I am no longer afraid to discipline my children. I want them to grow up to be honest, loving, responsible people. I know this will not happen if I don't give them consequences because I'm afraid they might not like me."

"I finally left my abusive marriage. It was very hard but I know now I don't deserve to be hurt. Staying in the marriage was not good for my husband either. It was like telling him it's alright to be abusive."

"When someone hurts my feelings now I tell them. It doesn't do anyone any good to have hidden hurts and resentments that just grow instead of being resolved."

Ignore the clamor of your ego screaming its survival messages in your ear. Listen to the wisdom of your spirit and learn to discipline your thoughts. Consciously focus your thoughts on living a spirit-centered life. The thoughts you choose to think create the way you experience life. Through prayer and meditation continually strengthen and deepen your connection with your Creator. It is within this connection that you will find the peace you have been seeking. To live in peace means living without fear, anger, resentment, bitterness, non-forgiveness, or any of the multitude of freedom robbing emotions which inhabit the ego. Peace lives in your spirit. I believe peace is ultimately what we are all striving for. Being the fallible people we are we often confuse the ego wants with the spiritual wants. Don't be discouraged when this happens just evaluate your motivations periodically to insure you are moving in the right direction.

I am not suggesting there is no purpose for our ego. Feeling pride and satisfaction in our accomplishments is not wrong. In fact in the world we live in we need a healthy ego to accomplish the task of providing the material necessities required to live. As long as we remember these are not the things that are the true substance of life, they are only the things that are necessary to sustain it.

"I have set my spirit free to learn and to explore. For everything I am now I will be so much more." Linda (age 12)

Personalize:

How is my ego-centered mentality showing up in my daily life?

_____

_____

_____

_____

_____

_____

_____

How could I increase spirit-centered living in my daily life.

There was a crooked man who walked a crooked mile
He found a crooked sixpence upon a crooked stile
He bought a crooked cat who caught a crooked mouse
And they all lived together in a little crooked house

The man, who was no longer crooked, had a good life. He had met many new friends and he looked them right in the eye when he said, "Hello, my name is Tom." Tom had learned to dream and some of his dreams had come true. He discovered he had many talents and skills. Tom had even painted his house, a bright sunny yellow that matched how happy he felt inside. Tom became a teacher. He taught his students things that couldn't be learned in books, how to see the beauty in the world and in each other. Tom could see the suffering in some of the children and he understood their pain and fear. He took extra time to show them, through his actions and his words that they were good. Each beautiful and special in their own way. He taught them they could dream too. Tom had learned these things through his own pain. He wished it had not been so but still he was grateful for what he knew. Grateful his own suffering had opened his eyes to the suffering of others. Grateful his heart was full of compassion instead of bitterness.

There was only one thing in Tom's life which still caused him distress. No matter how much success he had, Tom's father had never told him he was wrong, never said he was sorry. Sometimes in the middle of the night Tom thought of all he had suffered , all he had been robbed of by his father. Tom was filled with anger when he thought of these things. He felt again the frustration of the powerless child he had been. And even though he now knew his father's words were not true, he felt again the anguish of the child. Tom did not want to carry these feelings anymore so he decided it was time to talk to his father. Tom thought if he could make his father understand he would be sorry for the harm he had done. Perhaps then Tom could forgive him.

Tom was nervous when he spoke to his father. He remembered everything he learned from the doctor and he held onto it with all his might. Tom talked for a long time, telling of how hurt he had been, telling of how he had yearned for his father's love, of how much he had wanted his father to be proud of him. Tom told his father about the doctor and how hard he had worked to deal with the pain, how hard he had worked to build a good life. Finally Tom stopped talking, he had no more to say. He waited for his father to say he was sorry; he waited for his father to tell him he was loved. His father said nothing. He only stared at Tom with a hard look on his face. Tom could feel himself shrinking, he could feel his insides twisting, he could feel himself turning crooked. Tom saw in the man before him the powerful force that had beaten him down. He heard again the cruel words of his childhood and then he heard something else. The doctor's voice echoed in Tom's mind, "Your father was not a brave man. He lacked the courage to face his own pain so he passed it on to you. You must decide what you will do with that pain. Conquer it, or allow it to destroy you and others as your father did." Tom felt his spine straighten. He raised his eyes from the ground and looked at his father. Tom was amazed at what he saw, a miserable, bitter old man. A man who had never allowed himself to know the joy of love. A man who took power over others because he believed he had no real power of his own. A man who had spent his life imprisoned in his anger and resentment. Tom saw a small man, a weak man.

The anger and disappointment faded away and in their place he felt pity. Tom knew what his father had done was wrong. He could not forgive his father's actions but he could forgive him.

"I forgive you father," he said, and turning around he walked away. Tom knew it was over. There was no place left in him for anything that belonged to the abuse, there was no place left in him that belonged to the past. Tom was filled with the peace that comes from forgiveness. The forgiveness had come on its own. He had not needed his father's regret or his apology to make it happen. Tom wondered why he had not forgiven before. But even as the thought came into his mind the wisdom of his spirit gave him the answer. He had not been ready. Tom had needed to honor his anger, his fear and his disappointment. He had to face his father and tell him the truth. He knew his heart released those feelings at exactly the right time. He had set himself on this path the moment he decided he wanted to forgive. Forgiveness had changed Tom from being a survivor into a hero. For what can be more heroic than to look into the face of those who have hurt you and say, "I forgive you"

Tom climbed onto his shiny red bicycle, and like all good heroes, rode off into the sunset.

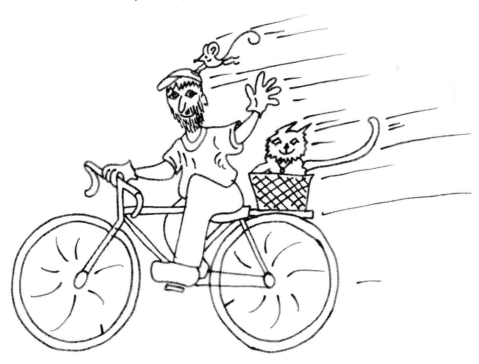

Bibliography/ Recommended Reading

Allender, D.B. (1990) *The Wounded Heart: Hope for Adult Victims of Childhood Sexual Abuse.* Colorado Springs, Colo.: Navpress

Barbach, L. & Geisinger, D. (1993). *Going the Distance: Finding and Keeping Lifelong Love.* New York, NY.: Penguin Group

Engle, Beverly (1989). *The Right to Innocence: Healing the Trauma of Childhood Sexual Abuse.* New York, NY.: Ballantine Books

Evans, Patricia (1996). *The Verbally Abusive Relationship: How to recognize it and how to respond to it.* Holbrook, MA.: Adams Media Corporation

Farmer, Steven, (1989). *Adult Children of Abusive Parents: A Healing Program for Those Who Have Been Physically, Sexually or Emotionally Abused.* New York, NY.: Ballantine Books

Hewitt, Fran & Les, (2003). *The Power of Focus for Women: How to Live the Life You Really Want.* Deerfield Beach, FL: Health Communications Inc.

Meyer, Joyce (1999). *How to Succeed at Being Yourself: Finding the Confidence to Fulfill Your Destiny.* Fenton, Missouri: Harrison House Inc.

Miller, Alice (1986). *Thou Shalt Not Be Aware: Society's Betrayal of the Child.* Scarborough, Ont.: The New American Library of Canada

Moschetta, Evelyn & Paul (1998). *The Marriage Spirit: Finding the Passion and Joy of Soul-Centered Love.* New York, NY.: Simon & Schuster

Muller, Wayne (1993). *Legacy of the Heart: The Spiritual Advantages of a Painful Childhood.* New York, NY.: Fireside, Simon & Schuster

Richardson, Cheryl (2002). *Stand Up For Your Life: A Practical Step-by-Step Plan To Build Inner Confidence And Personal Power.* New York, NY.: Free Press

Stone, Douglas:; Patton, Bruce; Heen, Sheila (1999). *Difficult Conversations;* New York, NY: Penguin Group

Warren, Rick (2002). *The Purpose Driven Life: What On Earth Am I Here For?* Grand Rapids, Michigan: Zondervan

If you have a comment or an inquiry you can email:
walkingthecrookedmile@telus.net

ISBN 141207542-4

Made in the USA
San Bernardino, CA
05 July 2015